WE'RE GOING TO LIVE FOREVER

THE SECRETS TO ETERNAL YOUTH

Ken Heathcote

Published by Ken Heathcote
Publishing partner: Paragon Publishing, Rothersthorpe
First published 2017
© Ken Heathcote 2017

ISBN 978-1-78222-527-0

Book design, layout and production management by Into Print
www.intoprint.net
+44 (0)1604 832149

Printed and bound in UK and USA by Lightning Source

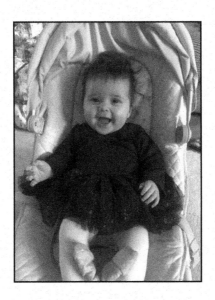

Dedicated to our
Great Granddaughter
Sophia Rose Thorpe
who listened to me when all of five months old, when the
conversation revolved around neuroplasticity: arms, legs,
eyes, body, head and a multitude of facial expressions calling
on all her senses to absorb everything around her. She gives us
hope, provides purpose, creates our destiny and challenges us
to find answers for the future.

CONTENTS

ACKNOWLEDGEMENTS

Thanking everyone who helped to shape this book would need another book twice the size of this one. Sixty odd years and tens of thousands of people who all helped to shape me, my life, my work and yes, my family. Someone once said that we are the sum total of our life's experiences and they are right.

In the early days of bypass surgery, heart transplants and micro-technology we had the local fitness people who were asked to help with the aftermath. Hundreds would knock on our doors in search of rehab and a controlled exercise environment. Athletes, soccer players and all and sundry: all helping to play their part in developing our experience of the human body and the psychology of it all. Where indeed do I start?

For this book, I start with the characters in it and the hundreds who do not get a mention: I thank you all. The family of Billy Leach, The Fitness League, and all who started the ball rolling with the local Fitness League at St Osmund's in Bolton. Jan Tate, from the same organisation, whose invitation to their course at Lilleshall changed the direction of the book. My special thanks to Ann Hunt who never shied away from volunteering information. James Hartnell who proofed and edited. Julia Page who typed and retyped. Judith Darby whose advice helped with the key chapter on People. My sounding boards: Val and Brian Whittle. Ted Wisedale whose photography nearly got him drowned. Also Tony Barry's blind faith in helping to promote the book despite having not seen it.

Last, but not least, thanks to my wife Brenda who has continued to suffer my idiosyncrasies for the past sixty years, or is it more?

FOREWORD

"The greatest discovery of my generation is that human beings can alter their lives by altering their attitude of mind."
— William James 1842-1910

PERCEPTION

René Magritte was a Belgian surrealist artist in the early part of the last century. He became well-known for a number of witty and thought-provoking images, often depicting ordinary objects in unusual settings. Many of his paintings, significantly from his work between 1918 and 1924, were influenced by futurism and from 1928 to 1929 he painted ‹This Is Not A Pipe' which is now on display in the Los Angeles County Museum of Art in California.

Under the heading: 'Treachery of Images', René Magritte›s painting shows a pipe. It is humorous in demonstrating that, yes indeed, it is not a pipe but the painting of a pipe. Magritte was a modernist, a surrealist, and if he were alive today he would be courted by the culture of today, via television, popular and classical music, fashion or anything that promoted image alongside reality. Many people when looking at his painting of a pipe will smile and ask the question: where does image perception and reality begin and end? What is it that shaped our lives, changed our minds and sometimes, yes, changes our life for a better future?

Perception and reality are subjects that have held a fascination for me since I started in business over fifty years ago. At the age of eighty-one, my vision was to write a book about growing into old age and still pursuing an active and vigorous life until the end. The book, I thought, would not be about longevity, only God can dictate that. No, it would be about being active. I had no title in mind, no plan other than food, exercise, the psychology of it all and something that revolved around community. These four subjects would be the cornerstone of the book. It was not long, however, before these perceptions changed and like Magritte's pipe, the image and the reality were so, so different.

REALITY

This book is about living longer and that is a reality. The people in this book demonstrate time and time again with their activity and their agility of both body and mind exactly what it means to grow older and still be in charge of both. The book was not going to be about longevity but now it is. One of my cornerstones, food, went straight out of the window. It was the people in the book that again changed my perception. Now, after six decades of training and exercise these seventy, eighty and ninety year olds would once again change my view of ageing.

'I'm not writing this book', I thought at one stage, 'They are!'

Not only do they have the wisdom, but they articulate it with some aplomb. All this and more would change the course of the book. Out went the myths on diet, the thoughts on exercise, even words like discipline, determination and the need to stick at it. Instead a word: 'stickiness' would emerge which meant the total opposite. A line or a word said in innocence would link with another line or word said with the same innocence a hundred miles apart, and the dots would need to be connected; and then the title of a chapter would find its place. With only a few weeks into my research, with myths destroyed, perceptions obliterated and my expertise in question, the whole book changed direction and out of the mouths of these ageing babes I was off discovering a new chapter in my life, and in theirs.

THE JOURNEY

I never saw it coming. How did dementia become part of the equation? Where did the word neuroplasticity come from? Neurons, synapses, pathways and brain cells: all language that had nothing to do with my research until Mary McDaid said that we teach both the left and right side of the brain. A brief conversation at Lilleshall sent me scuttling off to my notes on what someone had said about concentration. Then a book from the past, written and read in 1988 called 'The Healing Brain' and another modern one called 'The Brain That Changes Itself'' gave me much food for thought. Science and innocence merging, and yet another path to follow and another direction on a journey to find the secrets of eternal youth. People change their minds: they shape and influence direction, their words and thoughts challenge our own way of thinking, our own status quo, and so it was with this book of mine. Some will never change, not because they have no will, determination, ambition or belief, but because they cannot see a way out of the rut they are in. People just five miles from where I live will die on average ten years before the people in my location, not because of money, food or lack of education, but because of their environment.

'History', said one of our characters in this book, 'is important because history can tell us what works.'

Some of us are born into an environment of apathy and failure and are doomed to fail unless we are fortunate enough to lose the shackles of inheritance. For some, the journey will never begin, the reality of their past thwarting the perception

9

of their future. For the ones who escape there is a journey, a destination and a conclusion.

THE STEPS

The chapters of this book were shaped, formed and created by the people of this book. It never dawned on me that all these ageing stars were showing no hesitation when answering my questions. They were quick to voice an opinion, a theory or a particular thought. Many of them are still teaching well into their sixties and seventies. Strong in personality, firm with their explanations, specific in their judgement. I had little to do but listen, observe and interpret, and another chapter would emerge, another step, another clue, and another secret to eternal youth.

With each step came another clue, and the realisation that their minds were clear and thus the book took another turn. The primary target was not just about being active into old age but having your wits about you. Having got the comments of the present, these would resonate with the comments of the past and something that had been said over forty years ago would now make sense today. It is for this reason that I start with Billy Leach: his humour and his wisdom and his mantra will set the scene for the remaining chapters. The Fitness League is now over eighty years old and again this helps to start the journey. Both these chapters link us with the past and perhaps demonstrate the importance of attitudes. They were tough times in those early days with little of no knowledge of what to eat and what kind of exercise to do. These were the days of hard labour, ten hour working days and the Second World War. Many of the people lived to be in their nineties. Billy's attitude to food played a huge part in defining our chapter on the same subject. The Fitness League which started in 1932, was the inspiration for the title of this book. These women, like Billy, have always had a wonderful attitude to life.

What came out of these chapters is direction, and above all, the people's wisdom. Without their awareness, the chapters would not have evolved. It is because of this that Chapter 18: People, is in the near the middle of this book. I wanted them to speak to you, the reader. This is not a book about me, but about them. Yes, I relate some facts, some stories about me but in every case it is just to emphasise a point. I also feel that this is not about theory or academic study: I, like the people in this book, have been there, done it and as they say: 'bought the T-shirt'. Be lifted by these people, I certainly am, when coming across one of the characters flip to the chapter on People and see what they have to say, be absorbed and be inspired and in turn you too will aspire to be active, to be agile in mind and in body just as they are.

The first casualty of war, my Dad used to say, is the truth, and that applies to life and so it is with this book. Sixty years and more of experience, study, passion, trial and error have led to a final understanding that it is the people who in their wisdom will find the truth. This book is their story.

AUTHOR'S NOTE

The Fitness League used to be called The Women's League of Health and Beauty. Many still know it by that name. For the sake of this book I will refer to it as The Fitness League or The Women's League of Health and Beauty. This depends on who I was interviewing. The second change is in my reference to the neuroscientist Dr. Edward Taub's description of Exercise Constraint Induced Movement Therapy which I have taken the liberty of abbreviating for easier reading.

1 – BILLY

Carlton Walker stood in his sou'wester, waterproof mac and gumboots, clutching a spade. It was pouring with rain and Mr Walker, an entrepreneur from my own town of Bolton in Lancashire, England, was announcing to the press that this was going to be the best hotel complex in the country, and in 1969 he was right.

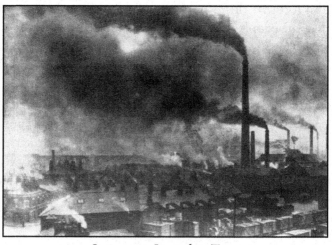

Smog over a Lancashire Town

The Last Drop Hotel is a custom-built complex consisting of hotel, conference centre, health spa, quaint old-style shops and motel-type bedrooms. The main feature of the development was a forty-foot panoramic window. The window looks over the town of Bolton and gazes on the mountain range known as the Pennines, forty miles away.

The Last Drop had been planned for the 1950s but because of smoke and fog, mainly from the cotton mills, coal mines and engineering factories, the development was postponed. It would take the Government's Clean Air Act of 1956 to signal the go-ahead ten years later, for Carlton Walker to build his Last Drop.

Slowly everything changed. The views became clearer, and parks, field and countryside in and around Bolton enjoyed a cleaner environment. The grime discolouring everything from buildings to clothes became a thing of the past. The population breathed cleaner air and no-one would appreciate this more than the long distance runner. Carlton Walker may have valued the views but Billy Leach, like all of his running colleagues, wallowed in the purity of the air.

I first met Billy at the home of the Bolton United Harriers. Leverhulme Park has a stadium with a circular track and an area for track and field, changing rooms and showers. The Harriers, as the club was commonly known, welcomed all athletes and was a platform for the wisdom, wit and psychology of a man I admired immensely. Bill was a miner for forty-four years. His knowledge of food was instinctive. His slogan was 'Health comes from within' and he lived by that mantra for over ninety years. His daughters: Sylvia and Anne, called him a Man of Iron. He loved his food but was frugal with amounts. Breakfast was porridge, sometimes with lemon and even barley. He loved fresh milk, eggs, liver and onions. He was a big water drinker long before it became fashionable. He avoided fried foods and everything that he ate was fresh. He rarely missed training and either ran or walked daily. His philosophy was regularity and when he went to club nights at the Harriers he mixed with his fellow runners, his colleagues, his tribe.

Billy Leach was ritualistic about both exercise and food but his greatest asset was his mentality. He really believed in the way he lived, the food that he ate, the self discipline, his exercise and above all his humour.

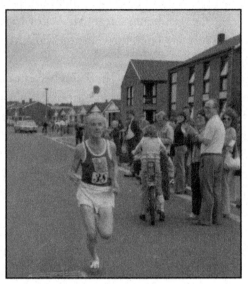

Billy Leach 1976, age 75

In 1976 I was asked to write a profile of Billy for the newsletter of Bolton United Harriers. Forty years later when I was interviewing his daughters: Anne and Sylvia, they handed me a copy of the article. There's nothing today that I could add that would describe Billy Leach better.

This is that article.

In the times of the Titanic, tramcars, trolley buses and tripe and onions, through the depression of the 20's, the First and Second World Wars, walking to work at 4 am to do a shift at 1,000 ft below, and then walking home, still with blackened face and body to bathe in the sink: in those days it could be all that, then a spin on the bike to the local weight-lifting club, then a run. It was not uncommon to do it all in one day for Bolton United Harrier, ageless athlete Billy Leach.

When the four-minute mile and man landing on the moon were still 30 years in the future, Billy would run, wrestle and do some agility work on the parallel bars. Clad in knee length shorts, long sleeved shirt and 'Woolworths Pumps', he would race over country, road and track, go home and in his own words...

'Have a yard o tripe fo mi' tay!'

'Thi mernt go runnin' o'er theer lad, tholes are a fut eigh'

Billy Leach's irrepressible and infectious personality impresses you probably more than the fact that he was born more than seventy years ago. When he talks, you are the target for a constant bombardment of stories from the past, anec-dotes, and a dialect and language that belongs to another age.

Laced with wit and humour, stories roll from his tongue. Like the time when he competed in the 'Fattorini Shield' – A three mile race at Moss Bank Park. He won in a record time of 15 minutes; a tremendous time, made even more remarkable by the fact that it was run on grass.

'If tha's never 'ad a puddin' done in rag, the's ner lived.'

He also tells of a challenge when bets flowed and colleagues said that a run starting at the Wagon and Horses at Kearsley (the slip road at the end of St Peters Way), going down Lord Street, Church Street, Cemetery Road and over the Red Bridge to the Nobb Inn, then back again, couldn't be done in 30 minutes. They still now talk of that event, and of how Billy did it. Not in 30 minutes, but in under 20 minutes. And of when he had completed the run a voice from the crowd shouted

"Now Billy, do you think you could beat Sydney Wooderson", and he replied in his typical and indomitable style:

'Course I could, but he's av come an' work down pit wi' mi' fo a month fust'.

I remember at Coventry when he had just turned seventy, and we were competing in the Veterans' World Championships. The over 70s age group was there for the taking, but Billy hadn't reckoned on the Swede 'Norden' who did a phenomenal 3.08 for the marathon. Billy's 3.28 got him second place. True to character, Billy couldn't let a performance like that go without comment and his immediate response and reply was

'E's ne'r dun it in that time, ther was two on um. One doin' fust alf and t'other doin' second.'

The year of the Coventry Marathon was a good year for Billy Leach. He won the British over 70s 10,000 metres and the Northern Counties Barnsley and Harwood Road Races. He also set a new over 70s record in the Barnsley Marathon.

'Am goint fo wum now and 'av a yard o' tripe fer mi tay'

Billy started running at the age of 23. He very quickly made a reputation for himself as an all-round sportsman: running, cycling, boxing, wrestling, and weight-lifting, and as Frank Morris, Chairman of Bolton United Harriers, once said of Billy:

"Perhaps the fact that he failed to specialise stopped him from achieving greater heights, but at least he enjoys the sport to the full!"

Nonetheless, Billy had a tremendous reputation locally as a runner and competed in every event from sprints to ultra distance. His longest race was the 48½ miles from Liverpool to Blackpool. Although the oldest competitor by ten years, he still came 9th overall, in a time of 6 hours 55 minutes. His performance in the 'Maxol' at the age of 65 was also outstanding: he recorded a time of 3 hours and 26 minutes, probably a British record for the over-65 age group at that time.

'Watch 'ow hi guz Kenny, durnt get thi weels fast int tram lines.'

Billy Leach survived the test of time. He completed many miles of running since those days of clogs, cloth caps and tram cars, when food was food ('If thas never 'ad a puddin' done in rag, thes ner lived.'), and nutrition was a word yet to be invented and before athletes 'competed' to win at all costs as opposed to participating as an escape from the poverty and grimness of the time.

We now have hot showers, changing rooms and, at last, Bolton United Harriers have a new club house, but Billy remembered when the car park at Leverhulme was a bowling green and 'after racin o'er park, wid go to pavilion and thid 'ose us down wi' cowd wata!'

If Billy can remember and survive all that, perhaps we should remind ourselves of the importance of athletes like Billy Leach in Bolton. He is our link with the past, our history, our heritage. He provided, for all those years, an example for us, and the youngsters of today may be the Billy Leaches of tomorrow. Youngsters like Mark Eastham, Paul Gildea, Richard Tomlinson and Andrew Selby. And in years to come, these boys may reflect on the days of Kenyon, Ovett and Coe, of petrol driven cars, sliced bread and fresh turkeys at Christmas. They will recall the running revolution of the 70's and 80's, rampaging youths at a game of football, the athletes who were paid huge sums of money to perform; and going back even further, they may remember this man who was from another age – a man who was given so little in life, but derived so much from it, a man who ran, wrestled and lifted weights, not for money or glory, but for the sheer enjoyment of it all. A man who lived well beyond the three score years and ten and still remained an athlete with the verve and enthusiasm of a youngster – a man who set those standards for you. So look to the future, but don't forget the past, and don't forget the name of BILLY LEACH.

Billy Leach was born on the 14th April 1906 and died aged 91 on the 13th January 1997. His death was accelerated by three things: a bad fall, ironically when walking down Wilsons Brow, a steep cobbled road leading to the River Irwell: because of the steep incline Billy tumbled and at 87 years old, this fall took its toll. Recovering from that to run again at the age of 88, he suffered the death of his wife Alice, but it was a chest infection that turned out to be the miner's cancer, silicosis, that caused his demise.

When interviewing his daughters Anne and Sylvia, I was privileged to share some of the moments of their father's life.

They said 'He died of a broken heart after Mum died.' Both knew that it was the miner's lungs that caused the damage.

The turn of the nineteenth century heralded the end of the Industrial Revolution. Billy, born in 1906, lived through two World Wars and over half a century of breathing the putrid air of his Lancashire Town of Bolton. I believe to this day that given different circumstances, Billy Leach could very well have lived to be over a hundred years of age.

Billy lived a structured life and followed a regime that included the essentials for a long and active life. He ate what we now call street food. Beef encased in a suet pastry, eggs in milk, broths made from vegetables; other meats like lamb, pigeon and chicken when available. His exercise was walking and running. He enjoyed the company of others, one of the keys we call Tribe. Billy's Tribes were his workmates, family and his fellow runners at Bolton United Harriers. He had a ritualistic approach to life, good habits to share – a clue to what this book is about and why he lived to be over ninety years of age, still active almost to the end.

In the forthcoming chapters we look at others who like Billy hold the secret to eternal youth. Their food, their habits, how they exercise, how they think and who their Tribes are.

2 – THE FITNESS LEAGUE

St Osmund's Church stands on the edge of a council estate two miles from the centre of Bolton. Built from red rustic brick, the church is a picture of peace and tranquility. Roses fill the small, well-tended garden. On the right is the shrine of the Virgin Mary and to the right of that is the vicarage. From the main road it is difficult to see the church hall which is obscured by trees and bushes.

Everything changes once I enter the door. The whole building seems to rock to the music of Heather Small, belting out the number 'Moving on up'. Ann Hunt leads the class and twenty-three women move as one to a well-choreographed routine of rather passive exercise. Laughter, like the music, fills the room and already I am drawn into the atmosphere. Everyone is laughing at some comment perhaps from their leader, Ann Hunt, for she too is joining in with the humour. I am invisible, they are totally absorbed and thoroughly enjoying their Thursday morning workout, and my introduction to the Fitness League, once called The Women's League of Health and Beauty, leaves me breathless.

This is no ordinary exercise class. For one thing the leader of the group is sixty-three years of age and just happens to be the daughter of the eldest, Doris, who just happens to be ninety-one years of age. Staggeringly, the average age of the class is seventy-four years, with a total age collectively of over 2000 years!

Welcome to Eternal Youth.

Having walked into the church hall of St Osmund's I felt two things simultaneously: one was that I felt at home, and two, that I had just been handed a bucketful of gold nuggets.

My early research had taken me to the longevity areas of the world, Okinawa, Sardinia, Nicoya in Costa Rica, the Greek Island of Icaria and Loma Linda in California. Now less than two miles from my front door I had found my fountain of youth.

I had never intended this to be a book on longevity: my early thoughts had been on staying active through old age. Now I was being faced by seventy, eighty and even ninety year olds who wanted to be active and not only that, wanted laughter in their lives, friendship and an exercise regime that avoided boredom and repetition and embraced variety. If I had just got that out of my research I would have been happy, but these bundles of energy and friendship had much more to offer. They, in their naivety, had hidden beneath the surface the true secrets of living longer and being active to the end.

My plan was to start with what nourished them. What secret diets did they have? It was obvious from the start that they were all in good condition, in that there were no signs of obesity, just a little natural thickening around the middle. I started with their eating habits and was more than surprised to find out how ordinary it all was. I was careful not to push them into the cliché of the modern and much fabled Mediterranean diets, the five a day or the latest food of the day. The interviews went like this:

'Just tell me what you eat on a day to day basis? Let's start with breakfast.' The answers came slowly, almost calculated.

'I usually start with porridge', was the most common (85%).

If it wasn't porridge, it would be either Weetabix or Shredded Wheat. Pause...

'And to drink?'

'Tea or coffee.'

Pause...

20

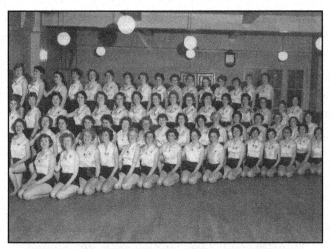

The Halesowen Women's League of Health and Beauty 1958. Lynn Ward's mother Wynne Barber was a member of this group (pictured on the third row, forth from the right) and 60 years later she is still a member of the League.

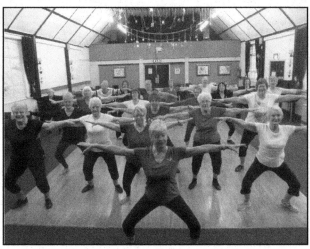

Ann Hunt leading the St Osmunds Fitness League class.

By the time I had interviewed the first dozen or so I was beginning to anticipate the answers. Lunch was always a sandwich: chicken or cheese or ham. Occasionally it might be fish - tuna or salmon. Almost without fail, the evening meal was meat and two veg. Fish was the most popular and again, chicken.

When I asked, Doris (Ann Hunt's mother), what she had for lunch she answered:

'I don't eat red meat.'

I hadn't asked her what she didn't have, so I said

'Is that because of the high uric acid or is it on ethical grounds?'

'Oh no!' she said, 'I just can't get my mouth around a pork chop these days.' Well, she is over ninety!

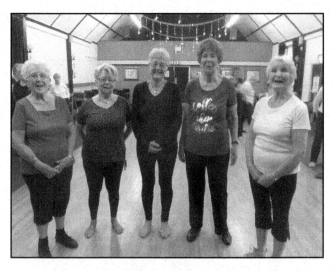

Long standing members of the St Osmund's Fitness League March 2017. Left to right: Mary Clare, Marian Berry, Lynn Ward, Sylvia Faucitt and Sheila Wells.

During the first eight weeks that I interviewed The Fitness League, I also travelled and interviewed individuals and other groups across the region. Only on the very rare occasion was I told that they followed the principle of the Mediterranean diet, the five a day of fruit and veg.

Derek Craynor, from Urmston, an eighty-eight year old bundle of energy, had Sugar Puffs or a jam butty for breakfast. Derek was training at the gym two days a week doing a mind-blowing programme all on a similar diet to the Women's League.

This group of people known as the Fitness League, people like Derek Craynor, and many more; surprised me by their ordinariness. The secret is that there is no secret when it comes to the food. They eat, but what was starting to emerge outside of the eating habits was a mentality that had a similarity to that of our friend Billy Leach.

'Moving on up', are the lyrics of Heather Small's song.

I was beginning to move on up from the ordinariness to discover the secrets of these ordinary people who have a genius for being active into old age.

After the first twelve weeks of looking and listening to these people, I was beginning to believe that there was something more than just turning up on a Thursday morning for exercise to music. For one thing they all ate the same food and apart from the porridge or a preference for a certain fish, they all ate just about the same each day.

I asked myself the question: 'Is this coincidental or is there some psychic message going on?'

This became more intriguing when I asked them what they valued most about the classes. It wasn't the exercise, they said, it was the friendship.

Almost everyone said exactly the same. And over 90% said the same when I asked them what they enjoyed the most:

'We have a good laugh.'

Others said they just liked being part of a group and they felt that history was important. The League had tradition. The answers to my open-ended questions were beginning to take on a different pattern and that was that they all said the same, without consulting each other.

I had made a point of interviewing each of them separately and they were answering me collectively. When writing my notes up later, I started to think that there was something more than just a group of people out to get fit. In fact it was beginning to look more psychological than physiological, more about group dynamics and even telepathy.

Social psychology studies on herd behaviour started in the mid-nineteenth century. Two scientists Gabriel Tarde and Gustave Le Bon, studied the mind of groups or mobs. Later Sigmund Freud and Wilfred Trotter wrote about this in their book 'Instinct of the Herd'. Malcolm Gladwell wrote about it in his book 'The Tipping Point'. Gladwell's book is about global epidemics and how they manifest themselves. One of the reasons that epidemics spread is in the social context that Gladwell called 'the power of the few', meaning that messages or rumours spread from just a small number of people.

There is a mentality that goes deeper when we become part of a tribe. Our instincts for self-preservation extend ever further when we sign up for a specific reason. The Herd of the Fitness League has a common goal – to be fitter. That is immediately logged into their psyche. Their eating habits are consciously and subconsciously exchanged, opinions on friendship and laughter are shared and over time they become as one.

The human race is driven by how we collectively follow. Anyone who has watched soccer will be drawn into the crowd's reaction to the game. All the players respond to the chanting of their fans. The value to the players is enormous: it's like having an extra man on the pitch, plus there is also the uncanny way of how the fans chant, sing or throw insults out to the opposing fans. All of this happens without any apparent leadership. There is no conductor, but the fans sing as one. There is no script, but they all sing to the same tune and the same words. This is what Freud called emotional glue, the invisible stuff that binds us together. When we get together, there is a silent understanding: no words are needed. The soccer fan just knows what comes next.

The herds of bison, zebra, buffalo, cattle or sheep operate thus. In psychology they call it decentralised decision-making, group wisdom or collective intelligence.

All of these things are intrinsic to The Fitness League. This is why it works, why there are so many who show the qualities of being active into old age. This explains the consistency of their eating habits through patterns and an ability to laugh and enjoy the same things at the same time.

Later in the book we will look at some of the other qualities associated with this phenomenon. We will also look at some other people from across the land, some of the secrets locked away in the lockers of their own minds and how they define a line that separates the culture from the cult.

3 – FEAR

Back in 1971 Philip Zimbardo, a Stamford psychology professor, set up an experiment that quickly went haywire. The idea was to see how people behave when in a position of power. The scene that Zimbardo used was a mock-up prison with mock-up guards and mock-up prisoners.

The experiment was to last two weeks but only lasted six days because the guards who were not really guards started to lose control. They became sadistic and showed very aggressive behaviour and the prisoners, who didn't know the guards were fake, became very depressed and showed signs of extreme stress.

This experiment was all about good people being put into bad situations and particularly how we all react to things that don't fit our expectations. The experiment was one of many and was probably due to a television show called Candid Camera which was all about putting people into compromising situations and seeing how they behaved and reacted.

Alan Funt, the creator of Candid Camera is remembered for some extraordinary scenes with his most famous one being called Face the Rear. The scene showed four people entering an elevator. Each of the four people, who have been told what to do, walk to each corner of the lift; but instead of facing the door they face the rear. This is when the unsuspecting fifth person walks into the elevator. Now we all know what we do when going into an elevator: yes, we turn to the door and this is exactly what our unsuspecting friend did. Like the guards and the inmates, our friend is out of sync with everyone in the lift and the pressure to conform is being challenged.

Slowly our friend starts to confirm first he turns his head, then inch by inch he edges his way around until he, like the other four, is facing the back of the elevator.

In psychology this is called mirroring. We adapt our body language to match other people under normal circumstances. When we go into a lift, we go to the available corners and turn to face the door – the exit – that is our escape. Another protective stance is to avoid eye contact. We are trapped in a small confined space with no windows and no way out once the lift is in motion. Our primal instincts seek protection. No one avoids this, we are looking to escape and our eyes move with the display panel to see what floor we are coming to. No one speaks because to speak not only takes us out of our comfort zone by talking to complete strangers, but exposes us to risk, and conformity reduces risk and risk creates fear.

THE FEAR OF SPEAKING

Glossophobia is the fear of public speaking or indeed speaking in general. The word glossophobia originates from the Greek words: glosses, tongue and phobia, fear and dread. There are literally thousands of phobias: the fear of spiders, of flying, of bullies, of being alone, of everything. All of these fears are self-manufactured except two: The fear of falling and the fear of noise.

These are the only two that are part of our DNA. It is not surprising that people fear changing their lives: being more healthy, eating better and taking up regular exercise. After spending over forty years of my life trying to persuade people to join our gym and health club, I was always faced with objections to overcome.

'Will I be able to afford it?'

'Will my spouse object?'

'Will I find the time?'

The fear of change is just as real as the fear of open spaces (agoraphobia) or the fear of closed spaces (claustrophobia), there is even a fear of fear itself and that's called phobophobia.

I WOULD RATHER DIE THAN DO THAT

Readers Digest is a magazine that has been around for nearly a hundred years. Founded in 1922 by DeWitt and Lila Bell Wallace, it informed and educated people on all subjects from health, food and culture to real life stories of courage and valour, to wildlife education and medical conditions. In fact anything and everything that would spark the interest of people would be covered in the pages of one of the most popular magazines of all time.

The Wallaces would also commission studies on many subjects from marketing businesses to neuroscience and even how people deal with the loss of hearing, or of loved ones or a debilitating illness. One of these studies was on fear and how people overcame their anxieties.

Part of that study was on what people feared most, which came up with some remarkable results. When asked what people feared most, the fear of death was surprisingly low in sixth place, behind spiders, heights and flying. In one of the studies it placed the fear of public speaking in the top three, which suggested that people would rather die than get up in front of an audience.

Although this would surprise many, there is a morsel of truth in that particular fear. I know so many people who have performed on stage for most of their lives who still become extremely nervous when performing in front of an audience. I have now been speaking in public for over fifty years and I still have vivid memories of my first attempt at standing before an audience and falling apart like a jibbering idiot. In fact I was jibbering long before I was introduced. So bad was I that I could not eat the customary meal that preceded the Farnworth Rotary lunch. I even found it immensely difficult just to hold the cup of tea: hands trembling, gut-wrenching and stuttering pre-talk conversation. In spite of all the weeks of preparation, the countless hours of writing my script, a life-time of study and practice about health and fitness, I still got it wrong on the day.

My performance was so pathetic I even forgot the opening words that said 'Mr Chairman, Mr President and members of the Round Table.'

And with that my host said out of the corner of his mouth 'It's the f'ing Rotary Club, you f'ing idiot!'

There is only one cure: get out and do it again!

Fear should be met head on and at nearly eighty- two and after years and years of speaking I can still remember those moments. I wish I could explain the reason. I wish that I had an answer that says do this or do that, practice this or rehearse that. There is really only one answer: face the fear and do it and expect failure in life and grow from it.

William Shakespeare's 'Fear no more the heat of the sun', says it all. What is so important that we cannot face that challenge? The exit from a place, the fear of failure, death, humiliation? The cold, cold water of a Lakeland swim, spiders, being alone, being with people or being without. The fear of dying and the fear of living. All make up the complexities of our inner demons that are just figments of our imagination.

WHEN MEN AND MOUNTAINS MEET

It was just before Christmas 2009 and the programme on television was celebrating the Daily Mirror Pride of Britain

Awards. I remember sitting there with tears rolling down my cheeks with the heroes of the men, women and children rightly being recognised for their extraordinary, selfless courage. When it came to our boys in Afghanistan, I was drawn to something that I thought was even more extraordinary. These stories were extremely touching but what really touched a nerve was not so much the squaddies, but the mothers of those boys who had lost their lives serving their country.

They were called the Band of Mothers, mothers who had put their grief on hold to help the survivors. The courage of these women for me had no parallel. There was no self pity. No blame and no reservations. They had lost their sons and daughters and stood up to be counted in supporting the other mothers' sons and daughters who were still out there risking their lives for them.

Watching this I knew that I had to do something for them. I immediately thought of our son, Paul, who had told me that he was going to climb a mountain in Switzerland called the Matterhorn. The saying goes, ' it seemed a good idea at the time', and that's exactly what it was. I was seventy-four years of age, and that good idea at the time would come back and bite me on the unmentionables. At seventy-four years of age I was about to start to learn another skill called mountaineering.

I had never climbed before in my life and it was fifty years since I had hiked doing my National Service in the fifties. The idea of climbing this iconic mountain was in a word crazy. Thankfully, it didn't come off because of heavy snow, but what did happen was that we climbed three other mountains with all three no less than ten thousand feet and all three vertical.

Fear and mountaineering are synonymous. The real kick that all experienced climbers have is the balls to overcome the fear. The best of climbers know that what they do is high risk and every precaution is taken but you cannot eliminate all the risks or the fear that goes with it.

The slogan on the T shirt says 'When men and mountains meet – great things happen'. I think it translated into 'You shit yourself!'

There is nothing more terrifying or more exhilarating than being on the rock face with nothing between you and the ground below. Your whole life is totally dependant on a bloody nail driven into a crack on the side of a mountain. We climbed something called a Via Ferrata, a safe climb by mountaineering standards. This is the side of a rock that has fixed rope pegs already secured in the crevices, steel ladders hanging by sky hooks it seemed to me, the ladders made from silver hooks and thin cables. The dots below look like a smattering of coal dust or soot but are in fact people. Reason, common sense, sanity and logic are now non-existent. The body, arms, legs and hands straining like the string of a bow, or a thread that defies gravity, not of the earth but of the mind; the moment that all climbers savour only when the challenge is accomplished and fear is mastered.

We were a team of four, none of us accomplished climbers, in fact novices, each of us learning by doing with only a modest amount of preparation.

FEAR IN BUSINESS: IGNORANCE AND BLISS

Working on a building site, climbing ladders, laying bricks or digging ditches is hardly the best preparation for starting a business. I remember that we needed money and naively didn't have a clue about how to get it. By chance one of he guys who came to my gym was an accountant and he suggested that I went to my bank to secure a loan. My bank at that time was the Old Yorkshire Penny Bank, so off I went, naively again or was it ignorance? The bank manager was called Mr Whitely and my request for money for a gym was met with laughter.

A little bit put off, I went back to my gym in the cellar and pondered the situation and eventually thought, 'What the hell, let's try it anyhow!'

The move to bigger premises meant a lot of work, without too much knowledge of what we were trying to do. By this time Bill Stevenson, my mate from the building trade, had come on board to help me with the alterations at the new premises. All that we had was an idea to make the gym pay. No business plan, no idea where the income would come from and no idea of costs. Even the best scenario was blind faith.

After the first year in the new premises, opening in just the evenings, we made a profit of just £50. We had taken nothing out of the business for wages, no expenses, and no money for reinvestment, and not really any plan or vision for the future.

Again by chance I had a conversation with the accountant. Note that I said the accountant, not my accountant. He suggested that I met with his bank, Barclays, and a meeting was set up.

For me this was just a meeting with another man. I had been told by the accountant that the bank manager would want to see a plan, some evidence that indicated how much money we would take. I had never heard of a business plan or what an invoice was or bill of sale, let alone a balance sheet or a profits and loss account. The only two things that I was sure of was that there were customers out there who wanted to work out and I would find a way of attracting them. Naively I had no fear that I would fail, so when Bill and I, along with the accountant, turned up at Barclays Bank, all that we were armed with was the guesstimate of how many members we could attract and how much they would pay.

I called this poor excuse for a business plan a 'Projection.' My business projection said that we would attract one hundred and fifty members and they would pay us £50 per year to train at our club. That amount totalled £7,500. We had some figures that showed expenses but very little else. Just how the bank manager totalled this up I don't know, but he came to the conclusion that he could lend us £7,000 provided he could have our homes as collateral.

This meant that both Bill and I, and indeed our families would risk our homes. Bill borrowed four hundred pounds off his mother in law and I borrowed the same from my Auntie Martha. Neither of our parents had anything. The fear of failure was non-existent. Ignorance is bliss.

In the first year of business, Bolton Health Studios gross takings amounted to £21,425. We charged a pound a week, cash over the counter. We had no substantial means of recording our income and our expenditure. It was a time when computers were the size of a house, there was no sign of mobile phones, no tracking systems for debt control, no statutory pay levels, no qualifications for people working in gyms, no methods of training people to slim, become fitter, gain or lose weight. We had no comparisons to work with in anything and we had no idea how to run a gym at a profit, because there were no gyms in business, because there was no-one in business running a gym that did it for money. It is said that courage is not the absence of fear but the overcoming of fear and for us it was neither: we just didn>t know.

Our business lasted for over thirty-five years. We started a business when the business of gyms didn't exist. We were an example of what enterprise is about. We were called entrepreneurs when we didn't know what the word entrepreneur meant. We started a business when there was no business, then pushed it along, pulled it along and started something that would grow into an industry. We developed training programmes and equipment that still exist today. We also developed systems and mechanisms that are still in existence today, albeit disguised. Aerobics was yet to be born; gym instruction didn't exist; no-one had thought of putting a beauty salon in a gym or a crèche; or a restaurant or squash courts or sauna and steam rooms. No-one had developed a philosophy of customer care or thought that women would embrace fitness, because fitness was just for athletes. There was no fear because we had no time for fear. There was no fear because we were young and oblivious to fear. We had no fear because fear was the enemy of progress and when the mind embraces progress then there is no room for fear.

1. PREPARE FOR ACTION
2. RED ON STAND AT THE DOOR
3. GREEN ON GO

Fred Davies was born within the sound of the Bow Bells; a cockney lad, tough, genial, and probably the most courageous man that I have ever met in all my eighty-two years of life.

Fred was a squaddie in the First Battalion, the Parachute Regiment. The year was 1954 and I had just been drafted down to Aldershot to take the pre-para course to see if I had the level of insanity for jumping out of airplanes. The pre-para course consists of punishing runs, mud assault courses and other courses that have walls to climb, rivers to cross and running over rough ground carrying a tree trunk; plus learning how to kill people. If that's not enough, you are expected to do parachute ground drills, mock parachute drills, real para- chute drills, drills that simulate exits and drills on how to use a bayonet on a scarecrow made of straw. There is a drill that rehearses the exit from a plane without the cumbersome kit bag that you would use when in combat. A kit bag carrying weapons, ammunition, blanket, water bottle and food. This drill teaches you to walk or shuffle in step, a discipline that is there to minimise mistakes when nerves are stretched to extremes, knowing that within seconds you will be expected to launch yourself into the void, oblivious of anything that resembles life on earth.

You are one man among another six hundred or so in space with just a canopy and some rigging lines, and your life totally depends on a static line functioning to open your chute. Fred, like me, could handle all of that except for one single thing and that was his feet saying goodbye to the fuselage of the plane.

Practice makes perfect, except that it doesn't. Perfect practice makes perfect but you can only practice jumping out of a plane by doing it. Fred would do all the simulation stuff without issue but when it came to the real deal, Fred's survival instincts, his fight or flee or freeze, would kick in and Fred would freeze at the door. In actual fact Fred didn't freeze at the door for his body, his chute, his ammo, blanket, food and weapon would leave the plane but his feet stayed put. You see Fred Davies was afraid of heights. When everything else said 'GO', Fred's feet said 'NO'.

The drill to exit the plane is designed to eliminate most of our fears. The order to prepare for action stimulates the squaddie to get busy. Check your chute, the bag, the man in front, the man behind. Check the hooks for the static line turn, right or left to the door, get into position, one foot forward, one foot behind in sequence. A choreographed shuffle, the mummy dragging its foot. Red on, the light that orders the final step for the front man to place his foot on the edge of the exit. The order, green on go, tells the lead man and all who follow to jump, feet first in the seated position, arms in front, a hundred and twenty feet, then jerk. All this happened to everyone in the stick except Fred's feet. Each of them sailing into space, except Fred, who tumbled then bounced along the fuselage.

The real courage of Fred Davies was in his ability to disregard his fear. Not once did he shy away from going out of the door. Every time Fred climbed a tower for a rehearsal of the jump, he would do it. Fred overcame his fear in all that he did and when his mind said 'No', he would still do it.

Fred Davies was one tough cookie: he was a scrapper, a warrior, a soldier. He was a man who conquered his fears; he just couldn't persuade his feet to join in the victory.

FEAR

Fear is present in all that we do. Fear in business. Fear in sport. Fear in life and the ultimate fear in battle. We have the fear of darkness that I experienced on more than one occasion when serving in Cyprus.

We were on patrol in the depth of the Trudos mountain range: it was my turn to take watch and we had taken a position on a narrow path that was frequently used by shepherds. We knew that the Eoka terrorists used this path, so we set up the ambush just in case they decided to come that way that night. My stint was 2 am to 4 am. The point was about forty feet from where the eight of us were camped. It was a cloudy night so we had very little light and visibility was about five or six feet. Suddenly there was movement and it was coming to me along the path.

The mind plays tricks when one is alone. Complete silence was a necessity. I was armed with a sten gun with an accuracy of no more than twenty feet. I had a round up the breach so there would be no sound from the gun. It was about an hour into my watch and I needed to move, but couldn't because the sound would magnify. Without any warning my right leg started to tremble, then shake uncontrollably. I felt no other reaction except that I could still control the gun. The movement was coming closer and I feared that I would give myself away. The other guys were sleeping and I had to make a choice.

Should I shoot?
Should I wait?
Who was it?
What was it?

I was trying to control the shaking: in the state that I was in, I would not have hit a barn door at five feet. There was no noise other than the movement in the path. No voices or dialogue. No heavy breathing. A steep mountain path at five thousand feet, a decision to make, a fear to overcome and an uncontrollable shake.

Suddenly and without warning the fear dispersed. The trembling stopped and my mind became clear. Without any hesitation I emptied the cartridge of bullets and then there was a thud and then the noise of a falling body, then nothing until the squad erupted into action. Pandemonium. The mountain side erupted with explosives, mess tins, weapons, scuffling feet, stone, rocks cascading around me. Fear surrounded me, panic, uncertainty and chaos lasting for just seconds before the training kicked in.

Dawn was two hours away: no-one could see anything until first light. There was no sign of a body or bodies. No living creature and no answer, except some blood on the path; even then just a few drops maybe from a donkey or some kind of animal but there had been no sound. Just a few moments in my life when I faced the fear of the unknown; I was twenty-one years of age and for the first time in my life I had seen into my soul and faced the uncontrollable fear that had no answer.

04 – CHANGE

THE LEARNING CURVE

Do you remember the first time you sat behind the wheel of a car? The thought of just having to drive it can be quite scary, can't it? The brain is confused because it's trying to cope with lots of things at the same time. Like moving your foot, the simplest of actions, but now you have to do it and move your hand to engage the gears. You feel uncoordinated because the brain can only cope with one thing at a time; your tutor is watching you and that adds to the pressure. Your spatial skills are going to be tested, challenged. What's in front? What's behind and on either side? You are conscious of feeling inadequate and incompetent.

Some areas of education refer to this as 'unconscious incompetence', the first stage of learning and the first stage of engaging your brain and your body simultaneously.

There are four stages of change.

The unconscious incompetence; meaning you don't know what you don't know.

- The second stage is when you know what you don't know, but now you are aware of it. This is called the conscious incompetence.
- If the process continues, you come to the third stage and that is called the conscious competence, in other words you are driving your car and thinking about it.
- The fourth stage is when you go into automatic mode and you drive across town without even thinking consciously about what you are doing. The final stage is called unconscious competence – auto pilot.

Growing up and constantly finding new ways to challenge yourself develop your abilities to cope. Change is part of life. If we don't look for new challenges then we slow our growth patterns and fail to develop our physical and mental capacity. Tony Ford, our case study, took up bowls at the age of 78. Not only did Tony learn a new skill, but he found his group of people who became his tribe. Who is to say that with the death of his wife would have started a decline? What we do know is that he started a growth pattern that enhanced his life. Tony not only began to play bowls, something he had never done before, but he met hundreds of other people who he never knew before. Tony is now eighty-four years of age. Six years of involvement and six years of growth.

Tony's case study is an example of what is going on all over the world. Researchers at the University of British Columbia have been studying physical activity and brain health. They commented on their results by saying that three aerobic sessions per week increases the hippocampus volume and helps to prevent Alzheimer's. Researcher Teresa Lu Ambrose Ph.D. said the relationship between physical activity and brain health is pretty robust and her research indicates that Tony Ford and the Fitness League, Derek Craynor and Mary McDaid are all in sync with studies across the world. Exercise combined with thinking challenges our brain patterns and those brain patterns or neuro pathways will not grow unless we actively grow them by challenging them.

Tony Ford, Derek Craynor, Mary McDaid, and all the people in this book have by accident or by design overcome their fear and changed their lifestyles. You can find out more in Chapter 18: People.

THE HALF LIFE OF FACTS

Samuel Arbesman, a mathematician at Harvard, has a theory that what we believe revolves around how long beliefs last before we stop believing facts. We used to believe that the world was flat until someone proved it was round. Cigarette smoking was once thought of as being healthy, so doctors prescribed them for relaxation. It was once thought that the moon was made of cheese and some believed that it had special powers and it would change people into werewolves. Well, I'm not sure about the werewolves but the other things, no. No-one ever believed that going for a walk would exercise our brains, but we do now.

Samuel Arbesman's new book 'The Half Life of Facts', says that everything changes with time. He goes on to say that until someone comes along and disputes something, it remains a fact. Mary McDaid's philosophy is that when her ladies do her classes they exercise the left side of the brain by trying to remember the moves, and when they are concentrating on their balance, posture and moving their feet to the beat of the music, they are exercising the right side of the brain. According to Mr Arbesman, science has now proved that people engage all parts of the brain, including the right side, the left and other cells across all parts of that seven pounds of grey matter. Both Mary and Samuel are right and so are all the ladies moving and thinking at the same time but there is another entity here and that is that our ladies are not just moving, but they are thinking about moving and for me that is the crucial core of theory. It's not just moving and it's not just thinking, but both of them together.

Both Arbesman and Mary recognise that the constant change of the choreographed classes forces the brain to stay active and build new pathways, but soon one gets to the point of half life and only then does Mary need to change and keep all the ladies' brains actively growing new cells and pathways.

RUNNING AND BEING

Dr George Sheehan was the guru of running in the seventies and eighties. His book 'Running and Being' was a book that captured the hearts of runners all over the world. 'Change is inevitable' was Sheehan's philosophy. Sheehan believed that running and being were one of the same and in his best selling book 'Dr Sheenan on Running', this is what he had to say on change:

'The experts may be right, stress can kill. Uneasiness of the heart leads to despair. Tensions do cause neurosis, but without them we remain in fear of our true selves. Forget the fire, the forge, and the flame; live if you like a life without risk, but remember the good things come in this tense restless and stressful life we live.'

Sheehan's analogy of the competitive race can be expressed through the many challenges we face in life. Stress, uneasiness of the heart, tensions and neurosis are all part of the commitment to the race. Without these challenges we will never know just how good or how bad we can be. Change tests us, change is risk, change commits but if we do not embrace this change then we cannot enjoy the real meaning of life.

Just about the time that George Sheehan was running and writing, we in our business of fitness were engaged in forging new concepts in working out. We only had backstreet, black iron gyms in those days and we took the risk of making the torture pleasant. All the emotions that Sheehan described in the run were pretty much the same with moving from a cellar and a back street to going above ground and changing the black iron to polished chrome. There were plenty of sleepless nights, not just for my partner, Bill Stevenson and myself, but for our wives and families and indeed the bank manager who gambled on this harebrained idea that we could turn a grotty hobby into a business. The ultimate result was Sheehan's line in that the good things that come in this tense and restless life we live go way beyond running and are a symptom of everyone's life regardless of what we do. Change is part of us all and change will never cease as long as we live. The business that started in 1968 has now morphed into a 60 billion pound industry worldwide and the changes that are happening now are reverting back to some semblance of fifty years ago. Free weights, barbells and dumbbells are even painted black; the design and decor are preferred to carpets and chrome, but essentially it has now changed back to what it was then. The real change however, is not in the equipment and the paintwork, but in the volumes of people and clubs. The two percent of people who wanted to work out then is now fourteen and membership worldwide is in the region of a hundred and fifty millions. Not such a big risk for the bank manager then.

Both Bill and myself had come from rather poor backgrounds. Opening a commercial gym in reality was a no brainer. What we had then would not make money in a thousand years, so it was obvious that we had to change something. Not knowing what that change was, we put our thinking caps on and brainstormed it. That led us down a path to nowhere. How can people conjure up dreams, concepts and tangible products if the dreams, the concept and the tangibility don't exist? What we didn't know was how ingenious the human brain can be and the two lads from the other side of the fence wouldn't let the brain stop dreaming.

It would take four years before the dream became a reality. Even then the change was still not obvious. We had moved from a four hundred square foot gym to a two thousand square foot studio and from there to a ten thousand square foot, four storey building. The strange thing was that it wasn't our dream or the concept that indicated the change but the size of the floor space that inspired the product that still prevails today.

A ten thousand square foot gym was still a no-goer. The problem we had was not the concept or the product, but what to do with the space.

To put a beauty salon alongside a black iron gym was ludicrous. A restaurant – silly! A crèche, sauna, exercise to music, plus steam and squash were all a change too far. History has now proved otherwise. The ten thousand square foot of space changed our way of thinking: a tangent, another path to follow and the face of fitness would change forever.

WHITE TRASH

'Hell or High Water' is a film directed by David Mackenzie. It stars Jeff Bridges, Ben Foster, Chris Pine and Gil Birmingham. The story is about two career criminals who rob banks to pay off the debt imposed by the banks that they have set out to rob. Chris Pine and Ben Foster play the two bank robbers in this modern day western. This cat and mouse story could easily be set with the James brothers a hundred years ago, except that Mackenzie's clever production tells the story through modern day society. The Sheriff (Jeff Bridges) is the one playing the cat and the two brothers Tanner and Toby (Ben Foster and Chris Pine) are the two who lock brains to avoid being gobbled up by the law.

Mackenzie's setting is central Texas, an area that harbours the so called white trash of America. This label signifies lower social class and degrading standards of living. The term has been adopted for people living on the fringes of the social order who are seen as dangerous because they may be criminal, unpredictable and without respect for authority, whether it be political, legal or moral. The term is usually a racial slur but may also be used self-referentially by working class whites to jokingly describe their origins or lifestyle.

This description of white trash is important to the theme of the film. Our two bank robbers really don't fit the profile of the underclass except for their homestead being reclaimed by the Central Bank of Texas. Mackenzie's illustration of poverty and hopelessness is reflected in the camera and the soul searching music, and in particular the attitudes of the cast who play the local sympathisers to the robbers. The story has been played many times from Robin Hood to the Great Train Robbers, but the sensitivity of Mackenzie's direction goes much deeper than the good guys and the bad guys.

I don't believe that Bill Stevenson and myself ever contemplated robbing a bank. We both came from the poor areas and if you were to retrace our heritage you would see how much poverty there was in the past. Bill lived in Kent Street, and that had a terrible reputation. I lived in a house that had no back door and because it was at the end of the street it went to a point. The builders presumably had run out of space and run out of bricks. Our coal shed was in the kitchen, a place to go when the bombs were dropping in World War II. Both of us could easily have been called white trash, but we were like millions of people trapped in a society that provided so few opportunities to what was then called the working class. Both Bill and myself crawled out of that rut when we took our gym out of the cellar. That one decision, that one crazy idea started a chain of events that saw a rather unpopular hobby become a business and the business became an industry that is now worth millions and we didn't ever need to rob a bank.

CULTURE AND CHARACTERS

John P Kotter is an academic at the world-respected Harvard Business School. His book 'Leading Change' is one of the best books of its kind on changing the concept of culture. The most important chapter in this book is called 'Urgency' and it had such an impact that he followed this book by writing another book called 'Urgency'. The theory behind this is that change will not happen unless we install the desire to make it happen. Everyone who contributes to this book, all the people who have been interviewed, showed a desire to be part of it: they all had a passion for what they do, often to the point of being too enthused by it all. In business it's called 'culture', in the individual and even in families it's called 'character', and this book is bursting at the seams with it.

When a business attempts to implement change it effectively changes its culture. This is very often described as 'the way we do things around here'. This book is not about the concept of business but it is about the concept of change for the individual.

In the case of the individual we call it character. If we wish to change, we also need to change the way we do things.

Being active into old age often means changing something. My wife, Brenda, played squash for years at our health club. Before that she played netball and rounders and worked out at a gym in Bolton called CAB Cashfords, and it was here that I first met her. Raising two children and supporting me through the big changes of our lives was not only a full time job, but a stressful one as well. Now at the age of 78 she plays bowls. She has found a substitute for all the things that absorbed her in the past. Not only that but it has also brought me into the picture for I go along to watch, not play, and I get involved in the social side of the game. One of us plays the game; both of us have found a tribe. The tribe furnishes us with a very active social life, charity get-togethers, cups of tea, a glass of wine, potato pie and peas and a group of people who enjoy each other company, share the fresh air and stay active into old age. I keep meeting people who are seventy, eight and ninety years of age. Like the Fitness League, they laugh a lot, joke a lot and probably eat a lot more than others but they certainly look good for it.

Brenda and her friend Margaret like the others have found a lifestyle that embraces exercise and a focus that absorbs them. It required meeting others, people they had never met before. It also meant a change of priorities, another thing to do along with her commitments to family, her time with her charity; Cancer Research, and the committee she works with. At seventy-eight years of age, Brenda has found a new dimension to her life, a new way of thinking, a sport that requires eye to hand coordination, walking the green and socialising with her peers, something that anyone can do if they are prepared to change.

An anomaly is described as a person or thing that is different from what is usual or not in agreement with something else and therefore not satisfactory.

We found change alien to our own safety. We are creatures divided by hesitation. Shall we or shall we not? The concept of change is either embraced or rejected by our thoughts. The fear of the unknown or the prospect of better things to come? Just growing older magnifies these images. Yes, we want change but have we time to rectify it if it doesn't work? I once asked a Major in the British Army why our soldiers were considered to be the best in the world and he said that at nineteen or twenty they had no concept of death. By the time they are twenty-seven or twenty-eight years of age that concept has gone, the fear of death then becomes a reality, so age and change are in conflict. But change we must. Dr George Sheehan saw change through the eyes of the runner. Forget the forge, the fire and the flame, but if we want a fulfilling life then we should embrace the challenge. Mackenzie's take on Hell and High Water saw his bank robbers risking everything to save the homestead, a legacy of their mother. John P Kotter's explanation came down to one word 'urgency'; for without it nothing will change. Both Bill and I and our families forced the change even if neither of us could see the future. Everything will change anyhow, said Professor Arbesman, because of the Half Facts of Life and the science of science.

Someone once said that our danger is not that we aim too high and fail, but that we aim too low and succeed. Aiming lower is less risky and aiming high invites rejection, not a great prospect in old age.

Now in my eighty-second year, I have committed to swim the length of Lake Windermere in the Great British Lakes. The challenge offers numerous risks. Until the day we won't know what the weather will be. Windy? Will the water be choppy? Cold?

Ten miles is a challenge at any age. The threat of infection high, the lack of stamina questionable. The heart, the mind and morale on the day – who knows. I remember at nineteen years of age volunteering for the Para Regiment: at that time I said it was for the pay. The miserable wages for national servicemen were less than £1.00 per week, but did it warrant throwing oneself out of a Dakota twin engine prop? The human mind is like no other. Why? How is it different, not from just the other species, but from our own colleagues, friends and everyone we know?

We can only change if we know what we can change to. We are all anomalies, each of us different from the next. What suits one will not suit others, so it is important to be ourselves for individuality is all that we have. We can only change what we can see, touch, hear or imagine: rarely can we change others, but we can influence that change.

5 – DESTINY

Coal mining in Lancashire goes back to Roman times. The coal seams were formed by the vegetation of tropical swamps and forests from a period known as the Carboniferous Period over three millions years ago. Tracing my family tree will only take me back to about five hundred years. I am sure that with some diligence that could take me back even further. It has become obvious however, that I have come from a family of miners. My Dad was a miner, my Dad's Dad was a miner, and my Dad's Dads' Dad was a miner. But Joe Heathcote vowed that his son would never go down the pit and I became a brickie. The year was 1950 and not only did I become a brickie but I also became a bodybuilder.

One of these two events would have a profound effect on my life. The other was just a passing uneventful period; almost forgotten in my eighty-one years of life. The tipping point, however, had little to do with being a brickie or a bodybuilder but everything to do with Dad buying me a set of weights. You see, the weights started a chain of events not about being a brickie or a bodybuilder but about organising a group of people around the set of weights. Without knowing it, I was starting to build my first club. I wouldn't be a miner or a brickie, but I would be a gym owner and the chain of events from that would seal my destiny. I would follow the road less travelled and the journey would last to the present day.

This is a story of things to come. The challenges of those former years have now changed: it is no longer just the gym, it is a place to go to meet friends, socialise, drink coffee, conserve and not just exercise our bodies, let off steam and either look good or feel good, but also a place to exercise our brain, develop the very thing that keeps us sane in later life and forges a future for our children's children and their children. Our mentality is now the new tomorrow.

It was Dad who broke the five hundred year chain. That set of weights that cost about twenty pounds would attract mates, friends of the family, neighbours. We worked out in the kitchen in winter and the back yard in summer. In the crudest possible way it became a club and it was the club that would shape the future. It would take years. The leisure industry was twenty years away. Our country was still reeling from the Second World War. There were whole streets of people without a car. One in a hundred houses had a phone, bath or indoor toilet. A shower? Something for the rich, but it was changing and with the change came better lifestyles, better food, and better education. The pits would go, the mills would go and the drudgery of life would go. We were a nation on the rise. A nation that would be healthier and yes, live longer!

Life in the fifties had an expectancy of three score years and ten. Now it's three score years and seventeen. We are beating cancer, heart disease and even diabetes. The challenge however is not about the body, but about the brain and the dying cells that are not being replaced. But for every brain there is a mind and it is the mind that controls the three and a half pounds of grey matter, and there lies our future.

Little did I realise at the start of this book that the people I was destined to meet would have the answer, or possible answer, to our future. Bewilderment and a lifetime of total absorption would change and with that the destiny of this book.

'You can't connect the dots looking forward', said Steve Jobs, 'you can only connect them looking backwards.' Sixty-six years were slowly changing with the people I was meeting.

'You have to trust that the dots will somehow connect in your future.' Jobs would go on to say.

Then I was with all these people, each one a dot. You have to trust something, your gut, destiny, life, karma. I knew that they had the answer but what? The thousands of people in a lifetime past and the hundred of the recent future would present me with a conundrum of dots and wisdom. The question: how do I connect them?

Who in their wisdom, naivety, practicality, innocence and instinct reveals their secret of eternal youth and vigorously living to the end?

Out of the mouths of sixty, seventy, eighty and ninety year old babes, we reveal their thoughts, the food they eat, their habits, exercise, and crucially the company they keep, and just what goes on in the depths of their minds. This story started over sixty years ago with trying to interpret what people think, what people wanted and how we could meet their needs. Sixty years ago it was all about the physical side of life, a smaller dress size, bigger and better muscle power, looking good on the beach. This was at a time when open heart surgery was being pioneered: heart transplants, bypass surgery. The challenges were enormous and the learning curve immensely satisfying. Sixty years on, the challenges are equally enormous but now the landscape is different. Now it's the brain, the three and a half pounds of grey matter, trillions of neurons and cells, synapses and the need to form new pathways; develop new cells to replace the ones being lost because of the ageing process: the New Frontier of medicine, a new age of exercise and a new challenge for everyone.

NEUROPLASTICITY

This is not a book about science, nor is it a book about medicine but it is a book about the new discovery of science and medicine called Neuroplasticity. Scientists now know that the brain can reinvent itself sometimes with the help of medicine, sometimes with the help of technology, and sometimes with the help of exercise. The information right now is not quite clear, a little like the information that we had some fifty or sixty years ago with heart disease. Nature however, has a way of finding solutions that previously we had never even thought about.

Neuroplasticity was first thought about in the late eighteen hundreds, so the last hundred and fifty years or so have been used to prove that it really does exist. We now know officially that we can develop new cells and even reverse the symptoms of strokes, brain traumas and even the effects of Alzheimer's, dementia and Parkinson's. What is even more remarkable is that we can now change the way our DNA works by changing our lifestyle, the way we think and behave, and how we develop new habits. After Dad bought me a set of weights and unwittingly changed the direction of my life, twenty years later I had the best health club in the country, a new lifestyle, new friends, a new outlook and importantly a mentality that our children would buy into.

One again, this is not a book about science: it is a book about people like Vic Trainor who went piranha fishing up the Amazon at 78 years of age. Derek Craynor who at eighty eight works out like a thirty year old; or the diminutive Eileen Mary Bailey who at eighty-three walks daily (eighty miles is nothing), cycles, line dances, swims and plays badminton. Or it could be John Higson who at ninety-five still does his daily exercise. Ordinary people living extraordinary lives.

THE SECRET TO ETERNAL YOUTH

We can't make this up. These people are extraordinary; they are here in our own back yards. Not only are they physically active, they are also mentally alert. In hundreds of such people I have found no evidence of dementia. This only struck me nine months into the study and the one to one conversations. For the past twelve months they came thick and fast, never dull and always surprising. I would discover an eighty-five year old class of exercise that is still keeping people active, creating friendship and as I would later find out, exercising their brains as well. This study came out of nowhere, a chance conversation with a class teacher in County Wicklow. Serendipity changing the direction of the book, and amazingly opening the door to a new discovery. I have been digging around all over the world for over six decades and here I am with buckets of gold nuggets less than two miles from my front door. 'I don't believe it' is the catchphrase of Victor Meldrew in the 1990's BBC comedy One Foot in the Grave, and neither do I but it's true and what is more, it gets even more mysterious. Get this... they are all eating the same food! These people are like the dots on a child's drawing book. Join the dots and you have a picture of a face or a whole body, a church, or a comic character, but this is no joke, each dot is a secret and the secret is to join the dots.

Simply bewildering.

Is this unique that I have found this secret? Well, I have to say no; the secrets are out there, they are in every town and city in the world; we have just not seen them. Take the food for example, every one of them or at least ninety-nine point nine percent are eating the same. How can that be? By some uncanny type of telepathy? Smoke signals? Like a viral influence of the mind? How can someone in Toronto eat just like our piranha catcher in Lancaster, or the late mountaineer in Switzerland eat the same as a teacher in Edinburgh; or the late Billy Leach have the same philosophy as eighty-eight year old Derek Craynor who lives in a tree-lined street in Manchester. How do we connect the dots?

DISCOVERING THE SECRETS

My old and valued friend Jim Halliday was a world-class weight lifter. Jim spent five years in a Japanese prisoner of war camp. Every day he would say he would treat it like it was the first day and the last.

'There were three things that kept us alive,' he told me, 'We had to find food at any cost, and we had to keep clean as disease and infection would kill in an instant.'

Jimmy came back from the notorious Burma Railroad weighing less than six stones. The food and keeping hygienically clean were extremely important, but it was the third thing, his mind that saw the end, that kept him alive.

'I knew', he said, 'that if I could see the end then I would survive.'

His vision was a muscular twelve stone middleweight holding a world record snatch above his head, six more stones, a medal around his neck, a smiling face and an arm raised in triumph.

Jim Halliday knew the value of vision. He knew all about focus and being in the zone. He would fulfil his thoughts; he would for a short time hold the world record in the two hands snatch. He would become the British Champion in three different weight divisions. He, like so many people in this book, was working class; he ate simple food, exercised daily and occupied his mind with concentrated effort. Jim Halliday practiced the habits and rituals and lived or died by how much purpose there was in his life, and by the power of his mind he travelled through time to the future. He learned the value of seeing the end first and worked daily to reach his goals.

Without a clue, I started this book at the age of eighty. There was no master plan and no title. I had no preconceived ideas, I just wanted to do a book on people living longer and being active until the end. To say that I was surprised is the understatement of my life, as the people in this book dictated the chapters, the content and the narrative. They have not yet told me how we join the dots. By their example, we have a formula. That formula is demonstrated through the characters, the chapters reveal the secrets. There is no beginning, nor is there an end, but perhaps we have come to the end of the beginning. There is no magic diet, nor is there any specific exercise but there is something that works the grey matter when engaging in our activities. The book will reveal how important friends, and being in the right company and the right place are for us. Be warned: convention is blown away. There are no fads or magic diets; it is so simple it's almost laughable, but it works and it has worked for the last eighty-five years.

The tone of this book is set in the first chapter on Billy Leach and the second on the Fitness League. Both these chapters take us back to the past but also set the scene for the future. Both chapters are oblivious to what we consider to be trendy yet they are not old-fashioned.

I didn't know when I started that this would affect our future. Why would I think about dementia? I knew the mind played a part, there is no-one more qualified here - just look at the record – but the book is not about me. It's about all these quite fascinating characters who have just knocked my socks off. Each and every one of them contributes to the overall answers, the secrets to their vigour in old age. So when you come to the chapter where I discovered the title, be prepared to go back to the past to learn the secret of our destiny.

Regardless of what we have now or where our future is going, what is important is the future of our young. Sophia Rose Thorpe is now six months old, so the work we do now is for her and her generation. She knows little of dementia or Alzheimer's; we know and we know that Sophia will in all probability live well past our life expectancy. Sophia's tiny little brain is at its peak in developing new brain cells. There is no other time in her whole life when she is more productive. I, like millions of others, would rather that she never needs to take medicine or find a cure for the debilitating diseases of the future. The natural evolution of our species will guarantee that some part of our existence has an impact on future generations. As always it will come down to just two things: the advancement of science and particular medicines, and how we look after ourselves. Personal management is demonstrated in this book. How we control our destiny, our future and particularly the quality of our lives is up to us.

JUST KEEP GOING

Each day, eighty-seven year old Len Russell makes his way to his local gym. There is a spring in his step, a liveliness about him that belies his age. His forty lengths of the pool is hardly text book swimming: he can't do the crawl because he doesn't have the skill. In fact he has never been a swimmer as such. He swims really because of a lack of alternatives. Len has had in the past four heart bypass surgeries, one stent installed, two knee replacements and major prostate surgery. His great redeeming feature, however, is his attitude because he just doesn't know how to give up. There is always an option, another choice, another reason to change, another form of activity.

Len Russell used to hike. Len like many of the characters in this book found himself alone when his wife died. His rambling was aborted when his knees were replaced. The four bypass surgeries demanded a more sedate approach, so swimming was a natural choice. His prostate and the stent are just inconveniences.

Why should life be a compromise? This seems to be his philosophy. Medicine sees him through, attitude keeps him going.

Len Russell is just one of the hundreds of people I have met on this particular journey. He is just one of the many people who help us to shape our future. Just as we are in the hands of medical science, we are also in charge of our own destiny, and the destiny of future generations. By studying the other people in this book you will see that there are patterns, clues and even definitive indicators of what we need to do to be vigorous in old age.

This book starts with the late Billy Leach. Cross reference Len Russell with Billy and later in the book look at Sylvia Faucitt. Then compare with Derek Craynor and John Higson, and Mary McDaid. Every time I write a name I create a dot and each chapter is a link in creating new ground for a longer and active lifestyle.

One of David Cameron's last initiatives before leaving office was to pledge money to find a cure for dementia. His reign gave way to Teresa May, but the initiative will continue. Governments across the world are desperate to find a cure for the diseases of the brain. The answers may not just be in the hands of science, but perhaps in the hands of the people in this book.

It was Winston Churchill who said at the end of the Second World War that this is not the end nor is it the beginning of the end. But perhaps it is the end of the beginning. Is this then the end of our beginning, are we now ready to forge a new future and are we ready to control our own destiny and look forward to finding answers to a brain that is just as active as our limbs?

There is no question in the minds of the people in this book who show so little evidence of failing memory. We know that physical activity helps in the prevention of heart disease and muscle wastage (sacrophenia) through weight training. We know that injuries, operations and physical accidents are treated with physiotherapy. We know that physical fitness is a path to physical sustainability. What we do not know is how effective we can be with building new pathways in our brains. We have always known that prevention is better than a cure.

6 – HABITS

SPECIFICS

The theory is that if you practice a specific change in your daily habits then you can change them forever. For over forty years I taught people the essentials of keeping fit and healthy. Our customers, a hundred thousand of them, all wanted to change. The changes for each individual ranged from losing weight, the number one request to shaping up, the number two request, to just getting fit, the number three request. Everyone wanted to change, but to change their weight, shape or level of fitness they had to change their habits and the habits they needed to change were everywhere but in the gym.

Our habits are our life and if we want to change that life then we have to change the way we live. Changing habits, however, can be quite demanding and often impossible because we are trying to reach into people's minds.

THE STORY OF DAVID

I once had a guy come to us to lose weight. It was pretty obvious that he wanted to lose weight because he weighed a little over twenty stone. One of our greatest assets at the health club was that we did a full screening on each customer which in those days really meant asking a lot of questions. There are several ways that we could do this, one being to ask open-ended questions.

We discovered a long time ago that we learned more by asking questions and particularly by what people didn't say. Sometimes this is called listening with the third ear. The answers don't always come in the early stages: very often, people don't know what the underlying reasons are. Very often, they don't know why they have put on weight in the first place, so getting to the source was often difficult.

It took me over three weeks to find the right button to press until I asked what his children thought. The answer I got had nothing to do with his kids' thoughts, but what he thought he wanted for his kids.

'I want to take them swimming', he said, 'but I am too embarrassed at this weight to go into the pool'.

The second thing that David wanted was to go in a shop and buy a suit off the peg. At twenty stone in weight, an impossible situation.

Once we had found his button we were then in a position to find ways of motivating him. So we made a habit of gently reminding him of what his goals were. Our habits helped David to change his habits. Three to four workouts at the gym and establishing a moderate eating plan, i.e. three meals a day and nothing in between and building up a rapport with our staff and his fellow customers. It is not one thing or two, or three but an environment that he feels comfortable in and a place to go that is part of his life. All of these things helped to change David's habits.

David lost over nine stone in weight. He worked out with us until we retired. When this happened he joined another health club and his weight was still the same twenty years after visiting us. David had changed his habits and the new habits became his habits of a lifetime.

BIG HABITS LITTLE HABITS

We all have habits. We get out of bed at the same time, eat and drink at the same time, park our car in the same place. If we go to the gym we will change at the same part of the place and often the same locker. We will probably use the same shower cubicle and sit and have coffee at the same table. We will go at the same time, leave at the same time; have breakfast, lunch and dinner at the same time: tea, coffee, beer, wine, water or milk. All fall into a pattern of habit. All these are a mixture of big or small habits. It would be easy to park your car in a different place or go to another place to change or another locker area; to sit at another table for coffee, and to change lots of other small habits. The big habits like eating less, cutting down on alcohol or stopping smoking, not over-spending or just getting out of bed an hour earlier are all much harder to break.

Taking up regular exercise or changing your eating habits can for some be a huge challenge so it is probably better to start with two or three small ones then when mastered go to one of the big ones. If it's losing weight or getting into a shape you're looking for then try to find some inspiration. A photo of someone you admire. If it's a smaller dress size, or if, like David, you set yourself a goal, keep that goal in your mind, picture it each day and see yourself smiling with your new image. Find a tribe that you feel comfortable with. Even share your thoughts with them. Don't underestimate how important the group of people you call your tribe is. Collective energy spreads: we feed from it. The feeling of security and confidence can have amazing results. Your environment is your stability, and stability breeds success.

HABITS AND ATTITUDES

Like everything else in life, it's our attitude that changes our habits. To change our destiny we need to change our habits and we start by thinking about it. The second step is to talk about it, the third to create the new habit and then to change our attitude which in turn changes our destiny.

THINK

TALK

HABIT

ATTITUDE

DESTINY

Changing habits when becoming old is more difficult than when we were young. We are more set in our ways, our thinking is staid, we tend to talk about the same subjects and find it difficult adjusting to the new things in life like technology, fashion and entertainment. Our habits are more entrenched, our priorities simple. Everything we need to do revolves around our desire to break the old habits and replace them with the new ones and that means attitude.

Thinking and talking will start the whole process. The phrase 'I talked myself into it' comes to mind. I remember going to watch the Great North Swim in 2014 and being overwhelmed by the sheer spectacle of it all. The atmosphere was electric with so many people enjoying the challenge of open water swimming. My thoughts were about all these people, different ages, fat, tall, short, thin and the attitude needed to overcome this fear of the mysterious open water. My reaction to all of this was that I should have a go at it. I wanted to be part of it, to be part of them and to share their experiences. It never occurred to me that the water might be too cold and that at seventy-eight years old, I would get cramp. My mind blanked out the thought of swimming for two hours in a lake in the countryside or the idea all the other swimmers would swim into me in the hustle and bustle of just getting round. No-one said at that point that I needed a wet suit, to swim in, or a hat or socks to prevent the cold. I didn't know that the water temperature would be about twelve or fourteen degrees, or that I had a two hundred mile round trip and a set time to begin and finish the event. The costs, organisation, entry fees, numbers, electronic tags and overcoming the fear were not even considered. I had already talked myself into being part of this huge colourful and spectacular event.

Looking for what you want to see is a great way of starting new habits. Talking to yourself and others is the second part of the process in forming new habits. Self talk, talking with friends, asking questions of others, all keep the start of a new habit in the forefront of your mind. The repetition develops into a new habit and by doing that discourages the old habit. See the new you. Visualise the new you. Talk to the new you and change yourself to the new habit.

For the last fifty years I have lived by the principle that every time we change our thoughts we change ourselves. The habits we create define us. They are our character and it's our character that creates our destiny.

HOPES, ASPIRATIONS AND SOME TLC

I only started to think about this book about a year ago and I guess that it was discovering the Fitness League that convinced me that I should have a go at writing a book like this. I know that there is a discipline required, a habit to be fed and a challenge to be met. I am not a writer in spite of writing five other books. It is not a natural habit, it is a forced discipline or it was until I started to write about ageing and activity. Putting pen to paper this time is different, not because I am better or worse at writing, but because for the first time in my life I am meeting so many people who want to share their life, their experiences and their habits with me. I have found a new world: just listening to these people has opened the door.. It has created new habits for me. For the first time in my life I have enjoyed the slog of writing a book. The exercise that I am doing now is opening my mind, creating new pathways and creating new ways of expressing the thoughts of others and myself. I am creating new habits and all because I am meeting all these wonderful people who want to share something with me. Their hopes and their aspirations are now mine because I care about them and they share and care about me. And I confess it's a habit that I am growing to like.

A NEW YEAR, A NEW DAY, A NEW YOU

The new addition to our family is now fourteen weeks old. Sophia Rose Thorpe is our first great granddaughter and is exquisitely formed, beautifully created and fun of unimaginable expressions and sounds of infant joy. She gurgles, smiles and even at this very early age, attempts to utter sounds that promise future expression. She now communicates, particularly when she wants attention. Her long periods of gurgling and silence are only interrupted when it's time to feed. It is only then that Sophia Rose is in the habit of grabbing her mother's attention. Her mother knows the nature of survival and so does Sophia. This is the first instinct, the first measurable sign, the first habit that ensures life. There will be many more habits to form, but this is the first. This is her first year and she will learn quickly.

The habit of eating and drinking will stay with her for the rest of her life: without food we die and we die sooner if we don't get food. The obsession with avoiding dehydration in these modern times started nearly fifty years ago. It was about this time that bottled water started to catch our imagination, when a study at the University of Sydney sparked an epidemic that still prevails today. We are consumed by consuming water out of plastic bottles.

One of the most common examples of this habit is no

more apparent than at a gym or health club, or with people out jogging on the street or country parks. People clutch their bottles far more than our tiny grandchild who somehow knows when to stop and even more so when she want some more. There are millions of dispensing machines that churn our billions of bottles per year, feeding the habit of dependence. There's water here, there's water there, there's water everywhere and most of it contained in plastic. How did our world survive for a million years without it?

One of the more extraordinary examples of such dependence is that of the football manager on television. Here we see the anxiety mode demonstrated with a plastic bottle, the misdirected plans or defensive error or a missed opportunity with a shot on goal. This is when hitting the bottle takes on a new dimension and the stamping of feet and hurling the bottle away is a demonstration of futility, anger and frustration. Everyone is hooked, both sides converge on the coaches, the physio, the assistant manager of teams when an injury stops play. Players from both sides rushing for advice and consultation and then it's drinks all round. Sometimes when the game is in its infancy, gum chewing, self inflicted water boarding gesticulations, arms, legs, behaviour that resembles the monkey enclosure at the zoo, are all there for the viewer and central to it all is the plastic bottle of water.

Competitive marathon runners will take three or four sips expelling 90% plus of energy over the 26.3 mile race. The ten thousand track or road runner will not dare to lose even a yard for the cost of a sip. The climber at fifteen or twenty thousand feet prefers tea or coffee and a square of chocolate; swimmers hardly drink at all, cyclists less than frequently. The jogger on the street however, will add to their already over weight frame, a bottle of the elixir of the mysterious substance called H_2O. Whatever happened to our natural capacity to judge?

Perhaps we should do as our great grandchild: she knows and she lets you know it.

Some habits, like unnecessary bottled water, are bad habits. The Fitness League, Derek Craynor, and the ninety-four year old John Higson, the boys and girls of the bowling club prefer a cup of tea, a glass of wine or a beer. They wouldn't be seen dead carrying a bottle of water across the green. Understandable if you're on a four hour game of tennis, or eighteen holes of golf, though even then the bar beckons, but carrying water is a habit we can do without.

GOOD AND BAD

It was Mahatma Gandhi who first said:
"Your beliefs become your thoughts
Your thoughts become your words
Your words become your actions
Your actions become your habits
Your habits become your values
Your values become your destiny."

Habits are a way of life, so we should cultivate them as we cultivate the soil. Each day in every way we can get better. The secret to good habits is the secret to eternal youth. Eat only what you need; drink only what you need. Take exercise or an activity that provides you with movement and especially movement that makes you think.

Practice daily the good things and the bad things will disappear. Find your tribe and be influenced by others, because they are the right people to be with. Make a habit of reading a little each day: it need not be much. Follow your dream to be active into old age. Read the case studies of this book and be inspired by them as I am. Love life because it's short and don't feel hatred for there is no time for hatred. Treasure the young and try to do good for them. Create these habits and do these forever because these are the secrets of eternal youth.

Good habits are reflected in good living and in the words of Joe Heathcote: 'Never wish your time away. Plan for the future and live in the moment.'

7 – RITUALS

The patterns had started to form during the fourth month of asking questions. The questions were all around the food and it had all become a little predictable.

'Just run me through your eating habits', I asked. 'Do you eat between meals? Breakfast, lunch, evening meals, what time is breakfast?' And on it went.

'We always eat the evening meal about 5:30 pm.'

'I have a certain way of doing things; I like to eat at a certain time, do my exercise at a certain time.'

'It is not just the keep fit; it's the company, the friendship.'

'I really don't come for the exercise so much as the ritual and the order of things.'

This is when I realised that there was a pattern to their daily routine and the word routine was part of their life. Routine is defined as a procedure, a pattern, drill, regime, a standard, regular, established, and natural. It was then that the word 'ritual' came into the conversation.

I must have met a little over a hundred people before I realised that everyone who I was interviewing was ritualistic in their actions. They wanted that discipline in their lives. They embraced the conscious effort to go to wherever it was to get their daily fix of company, friendship, enjoyment and exercise. Ritual, by definition is a belief in something that provides and order to our lives, something to be done that is not necessarily pleasurable, but is thought to be worthwhile and valued for its contribution to their lifestyle.

In October 2016 The Telegraph ran an article on a British runner who now lives in Canada. Ed Whitlock was eighty-five years old at the time and he had just completed the Toronto

Waterfoot Marathon in 3 hours 56 minutes and 33 seconds. Overnight Ed Whitlock became world famous.

Ed typifies the endurance athlete. He confesses to be being competitive; he also says that training can be a drag. In addition, he says that running provides him with solitude which he values highly. He thinks nothing of running three hours in the vast area of the Toronto Cemetery. Ed just loves to run even if it can be a drag. Ed, like Derek Craynor who is now eighty-nine years of age, loves his demanding workouts. Like Sylvia Faucitt and all the women of the Fitness League, they value the commitment and the need to fill their lives with something that demands that discipline and ritual. John Higson, who is ninety-four, exercises daily, walks and follows a ritual to fulfil an obligation, not to others but to himself. Ulrich Inderbinen, like Ed Whitlock, lived his life around his daily hikes. Inderbinen walked and climbed the mountains of his home in Switzerland until he was over a hundred years old. Like Ed, Derek, John and all the others, he needed something besides just living.

Ritual, unlike habit, is dependent on conscious thought. It is a part of our lives and eases us through the stresses and strains that challenge our existence. Religion, war, medicine, law, business, family and sport all have a place for ritual. All religions are based on ceremonial rituals, the soulless drills ensure automatic action. There is a ritual and process when conducting the smallest of operations. Solicitors, lawyers and barristers are bound by policies, procedures and disciplines that leave no room for error. Only through ritual do we protect the status quo and this is most evident in the performance of sport.

Back in 1981 David Puttnam, the film producer, told the historical story of two young athletes who were representing Britain in the 1924 Olympic Games in Paris. The two athletes both competed in the sprint events: Eric Liddell ran in the one hundred yards and Harold Abrahams in the four hundred yards. The story written by Colin Welland was a smorgasbord of mixed metaphors: politics, power, religion and race. Eric Liddell was a devout Scottish Christian and Abrahams an English Jew who ran to overcome prejudice. The film was nominated for seven academy awards; one of them being the music of Vangelis, that won the award for best original score.

Although the film puts great emphasis on the political and religious aspects, it is the portrayal of the athletes' desire to win that makes the film so outstanding. Colin Welland's script is masterful in capturing the emotions and ritualistic approach to competing and in particular to winning. Liddell is chastised by his sister for running when he should be praying and attending church. Abrahams employs a coach, Sam Mussabini, a practice that was not allowed in the days of pure amateurism. The Olympic Committee is made up of politicians, businessmen and would be representatives of the athletes; they are displayed has cigar smoking, brandy drinking aristocrats manipulating the sport for prestige (Abrahams was a student of Cambridge) and political superiority. All this is handled supremely by Puttnam. A wonderful film made better by Welland's understanding of the athletes.

Doubts insinuate emotional conflict and pressures of all kinds into the minds of both the runners, separating the world from the event. But having a ritual of preparation is one of the most powerful tools in every athlete's locker. The scene is set to Vangelis's music and the process of reaching the starting line starts in the mind with a well-practiced choreography of movement.

The eyes scan the changing room on entry. Who's who? Who is doing what? How is the opposition assessed? The sequence of undress starts and finishes exactly the same for every event: shoes come out of the bag first, then the singlet and shorts, a purposeful, conscious, methodical system of separating thought from action. Like the preamble to the race, the musical background is almost unnoticeable but our senses are starting, like the athletes, to slowly respond to what lies ahead. The audience, like the players on the stage, is there in the minds of the runners; only ritual can detach the emotion from the tension developed by intense competition.

None of this is new. Each week we can watch sport on television. We can witness soccer players, rugby players and competitors at the very highest level warming up. What we don't see is what pre-empts the start of our entertainment. Sport is riddled with superstitions and fears and they inform the ritual. David Beckham confessed to placing drinks in line before the game. I have known hundreds of soccer players who cannot start a game without following a meaningless ritual. Paul Ince would never put his shirt on before leaving the tunnel. World class basketball player Michael Jordan always wore his North Carolina College shorts under his Chicago Bulls uniform and a soccer friend of mine would never draw his bedroom curtains the night before a game.

The opposite to attention is distraction. All the rituals we need are always of our own design to get into the right frame of mind to do what we want or need to do. Joe Heathcote had it, Billy Leach had it; certainly the likes of Jonah Barrington, Bill Pearl and a friend of mine called Roger Bourban had it.

Roger, a restaurateur from Beverly Hills in Los Angeles, developed a skill for running while carrying a tray complete with wine. He did this in all his races, even the marathon. In the London Marathon, Roger achieved a time of 2:41:0. He was dressed in his waiter's uniform complete with tie, his tray was complete with a bottle of wine and this ritual served him well for well over ten years of running. Even with all the distraction of his gimmick, Roger could still run at a high level. Mary McDaid, in County Wicklow, had her rituals and when she said that we develop the brain through exercise, she confirmed it by showing its significance in her life. Ritual is all about believing that the discipline is worth it. All of these people, and perhaps everybody in this book, know that having a sense of ritual helps to drive us forward. The difficulty is not learning from the past or believing in the present but what we are preparing for the future.

TIME

Our friends from Oregon, Bill and Judy Pearl, live on their homestead just a stone's throw from the legendary Oregon Trail, a much favoured landscape for western film producers. Bill and Judy are both ardent trainers and open their 'Barn' to anyone who wishes to join them at 6 am each morning. Bill, of course, is just as big a legend as the Oregon Trail, with his iconic status in bodybuilding. People from all over the area of Talent, their nearest town, have trained with Bill and Judy for decades, always rising in the early hours for their daily ritual.

The 'Barn' is the gym, a thousand square foot retreat, crammed with the latest equipment for strength, shape and fitness. To workout with the Pearls is not a chore, but a privilege, even at 6 am. Outside of that very exclusive group of people (about 100), few will know that Bill and Judy's ritual does not actually start at 6 am, but at 3 or 4 am. Their principle, like mine, is if you want to do something that you value then you make the time. Bill's philosophy in life is contained in one of his best selling books: "Keys to the Inner Universe". One famous quote from it says:

'Now is not the time. The time is now.'

When Bill was asked at a conference in Chicago, why he

trained at 3 am, he answered to the young female reporter:

'What else is there to do at 3 am in the morning?'

Bill and Judy Pearl are similar to many great people in history: fitting their valued rituals around their busy days is not so much based on what they like but on finding a place in life to like what they do. Changing that mentality is all about overcoming the obstacles in life.

So many great people have embraced that philosophy. Time is short. Franz Kafka, the legendary 20th century author, said that life is never straightforward, one must wriggle through. Franz would start his creative work at 10:30 pm working through to the early hours. T S Eliot was the same, working and creating his poetry and his books between his hours of work at a local bank. Tchaikovsky's ritual was a two hour walk every day, timed to exactly one hundred and twenty minutes. The great female writer Patricia Highsmith's ritual was to eat exactly the same food each and every day.

William James, the progenitor of modern psychology, best articulated the mechanism by which a strict routine might help unleash the imagination in saying that only by rendering many aspects of life automatic and habitual could we free our minds to advance to really interesting fields of action.

Ernest Hemingway approached writing like sex.

'*You write until you come to a place where you still have your juice and you know what will happen next and you stop and try to live through until the next day when you hit it again. You have started at six in the morning say, and may go on until noon or be through before that, when you stop you are empty, and at the same time full; as when you have made love to someone who you love. Nothing can hurt you, nothing can happen, nothing means anything until the next day when you do it again. It is the wait until the next day that is hard to get through. Tough job this writing.*' (from The Paris Review 1958)

Beethoven, Winston Churchill, Emmeline Pankhurst, and Margaret Thatcher all had their rituals. Acting genius Meryl Streep has developed a ritualistic approach to living the part of her latest character for every part she plays.

Regardless of the lifestyle, ritual plays a significant part in helping us to get where we want to go. When meeting the hundreds of people from the Fitness League I was struck by how it is synonymous with military drills. The genius of Mary Baggott Stack, the founder of the Women's League of Health and Beauty, lay in combining the systems and strict adherence to its principle with humour, friendliness and sheer enjoyment. This did not happen by accident. Ritual is not perceived as being light hearted nor is the military delivery of perfectly rehearsed movement but the blend is obvious. She not only had a vision to build an empire of fitness and beauty, but had the ambition to drive a philosophy of fun at the same time. Ritual, 'a religious or solemn ceremony consisting of a series of actions performed according to a prescribed order', is the Fitness League to a tee, except that the dictionary forgot to mention friendship, fun and living a life to the end.

HOW

In August 2017, I shall swim the full length of Lake Windermere in the Lake District. My decision was based on two reasons. One, it offered me a challenge that needed a great deal of preparation and a mind focused on one single event. The second reason was that anything that is so demanding heightens my desire for life. The decision to do it hinged on whether I felt it doable. If it's not doable then it is useless to even try. Climbing Mount Everest is not doable at eighty-two, nor is trekking to the South or North Pole. Abseiling down the Shard is possible and I have thought of that, but dismissed it, not because I didn't want to but because the lake swim just seemed better at this time.

I had two reasons but in fact there are three rules. Having something to focus on is the first rule when we enhance our lives. This can be anything from getting in shape, losing a stone in weight, running a half marathon, or a marathon or indeed doing anything that will test you or bring something into your life that generates a sense of fulfilment. When we went to climb the Matterhorn in Switzerland in 2012, we could not get into the climb because of heavy snow, but we still found other climbs that tested our nerve and sinew and the vertical climbs left us, or should I say me, exhausted but fulfilled and immensely satisfied. So the second rule is to find something that gives your ego a boost - the feel good factor. We need these things in life because life is for living and without testing yourself then how do you know that you have lived a life?

In the book "The Revenant", Hugh Glass, a hunter in the early west of the United States was mauled by a grizzly bear. The story by Michael Punke, was made into a successful film staring Leonardo DiCaprio and tells the story of how Glass (DiCaprio) dragged himself over 200 miles to seek revenge on the men who left him to die alone. Punke's book and the film centre around Glass's epic and impossible journey, over-coming crippling injuries, near death experiences, starvation, attacks from marauding Native American Indians and the constant battle with the harsh uncompromising environment of the snow-covered mountains. The true story, or a story based on truth, is a triumph over adversity, a tale of impossible odds and a man's determination to overcome them. The book and the film are just an example of so many stories of how people can find a way when all the odds are stacked up against them.

The third rule is to just do it. This is life: if it fails it fails, but get on with it.

Joe Heathcote was a fine example of resilience. At the age of thirty-four, Joe was the casualty of a mining accident. My recollection of that period was that times were tough and really that was it: something to get over. Dad eventually recovered enough to function: at thirty-four he had his life in front of him; he also had two kids and a wife to support. Like Hugh Glass, he had to find a way. Dad's way was to keep going, follow the rules, keep your head down and do what you know best. Dad's survival, and his adherence to the ritual of regular exercise was expressed in the local swimming baths. I am sure now that Dad's philosophy (he wouldn't have used that word) was 'Just keep going, don't ask too many questions of yourself and focus on the present'. Both Hugh Glass and Joe Heathcote did exactly that: live life now. Both of them had a goal and both just kept trying.

Dad's resilience kept him alive, but twenty-four years later he would be tested again. At fifty-eight years of age he had a massive heart attack. Once more he was at death's door. Once more he would have a battle first to survive, then to live and, more importantly, get back into his old regime and the rituals that gave him so much strength.

Not for one minute do I believe that this resilience is restricted to the few. All of us have this inner strength: we had it in the war when the country survived the Blitz and before that with poverty, the under classes living through the industrial age and the First World War. The human race is designed to fight, to claw its way out, whatever that out is. We are made and put together to find ways to overcome, to do what we need to do - that sense of pride. We found it through the ages, through the poverty and through the two world wars. We found it again with our troops in Afghanistan. We found it by running in the London Marathon or all the marathons and park runs, triathlons, or anything that provides focus, challenge and the will to do it. All of these events and unexpected challenges make up the substance of who we are.

Hugh Glass died some years after his epic journey across the mountains of the Wild West. Joe Heathcote lived until he was ninety-seven years of age. His last thirty-five years he lived with angina. It didn't stop him following his rituals of swimming, lifting weights or going for long walks.

For the past seventy years I have lived with this subject: part of my education and experience was and still is living with people who set us our examples. Dad was practicing the philosophy of these people: Billy Leach, John Higson, Ed Whitlock, Bill Pearl, Ann Hunt and her mother Doris, Lynn Briggs, Sylvia Faucitt, Mary McDaid and Derek Craynor, all of them telling us something that we need to embrace. Focus, find a way and just do it. These are the strategies that we need along with the rituals that sustain them.

8 – TRIBE

TRIBE:
A social division in a traditional society consisting of families or communities linked by a social, economic, religious or blood ties, with a common culture and dialect, typically having a recognised leader.

HERD:
A large group of mammals living and feeding together; especially a group of cattle, sheep etc.

The definition of TRIBE is of a group of people who think together and act together. The definition of HERD is associated with a group of animals that act by instinct.

TRIBE

Probably the most in-depth tribe study of recent times is told through the chronicles of Brexit. A country, or indeed a continent separated by a single vote. The one and only question was to leave or to stay. Here we had a tribe of sixty million with one half wanting to stay and be part of the bigger tribe and the other half prepared to go it alone and risk losing the protection of the many and the security of the mass. The Daily Telegraph described one side as the white collar working class, the older generation, the survivors of wars and decisions made for them to be sent to the front line of the First World War, to the Somme and the slaughter of millions and a history of not being considered. Rightly or wrongly it was one half of a nation at last who had a chance to say yea or nay.

The world is divided by opinions: we as human beings

make decisions and this is ultimately better than instinct alone in our fight to survive.

Since the beginning of time we have sought safety by herding together to protect ourselves from threat. The tribes we use are our way of surviving these threats. The choices are our only way forward in our day to day existence. Our choices are crucial. Our friends, our families, our tribes are crucial, and it is crucial that we surround ourselves with people we trust, enjoy and respect.

This book is about surviving longer and being in a stable, functioning condition to the end. To do this we should take care to have the right people around us. The people who are 'armed' and provide us with the tools we need in order to live. We need to survive physically, emotionally, spiritually and collectively. Being alone in this world is not an option if we are to grow older and still be independent to the end. We need to be supported by others whilst building and sustaining life.

We are by design social creatures. It is not by accident that we herd together for protection. This social interaction is there for a reason. We network to learn and prosper and do this in the company of others. We express our opinions sometimes controversially. The Brexit vote to leave is a prime example of emotion overcoming logic with the older generation expressing their frustration at being governed by a much bigger and detached force that by its detachment ignored the fundamental feelings of the herd. Perhaps we are safer, stronger and more stable with a larger herd but unless the head conveys that to the heart our emotions will make the decisions.

THE HEAD AND THE HEART

We are all sheep until we decide. Only when we make conscious decisions do we separate ourselves from the animals of this planet. An example of this was the research led by Jens Krause PhD, of Leeds University. Krause performed an experiment with a group of people who were assembled in a large hall. The participants were told simply to walk around the hall but not talk to each other. Ninety-five per cent were unaware that a minority had been directed to split and walk around in different directions. Every one of the uninformed people followed the informed - they followed the five per cent.

'There are strong parallels with animal behaviour', says Professor Krause, who reports the work with John Dyer in the journal Animal Behaviour with colleagues from the Universities of Oxford and Bangor.

All of us have been in situations where we get swept along with the crowd, but what is interesting about this research is that our participants ended up making a conscious decision, despite the fact that they weren't allowed to talk or gesticulate to one another. In most cases the participants didn't realise that they were being led by others.

The work follows another study by Dr Simon Reader of Utrecht University, which shows that most of us are happy to play 'follow my leader' even if we know that the others don't know where they are going. What is even more striking is that this study also found that when we are shown a faster route, we will still follow the leader but tell the others about the faster route.

The difference between herd and tribe is that the herd has no head and is without the heart. Krause and his team simply took the head away and left it to be led by the five per cent, not unlike the European Market. Yes, the herd is fed and moves from grazing ground to grazing ground and the herd will find water to survive but will have no emotional urge to explore, be curious or expand its basic instincts. The herd, like the people in the hall, will simply drift and go with the flow. The difference between the tribe and the herd is simple: one is led by thought, the other by instinct. One is reliant on emotion, the other by the actions of the mass. The herd is without leadership and the tribe is dependent on leadership. The herd drifts; the tribe is driven by purpose, direction and accomplishment.

In 1968 my partner Bill Stevenson and I started a business called Bolton Health Studio. A health studio was a posh name for a gym. All other gyms across the world were equipped with weights and not much else and in 1967 that was all we had. We, like millions across the world, were training and pumping iron in places like school halls and disused premises that had seen better days. Our attempt at running a gym was in a cellar; above it was a shop called Maxwell Jones that sold typewriters. I think we paid about ten shillings a week rent. The cellar was seventeen feet long and twelve feet across. There were just two light bulbs and the walls were whitewashed. We had no running water and no changing rooms. Significantly we had no women, not a single female trainer and who could blame them!

Moving out and finding a place where we could express ourselves was a move that depended on luck rather than judgement. Nevertheless we moved to pastures new. Within four years we had developed a club that was unparalleled in the business of keeping fit.

The first thing we did was to implement just three things which we called it the three C's: chrome, carpets and conifers.

We built a restaurant in the club, showers, lockers and a sauna. We had a crèche and a beauty salon and we found space to run exercise classes to music, a concept copied from the Women's League of Health and Beauty. We had something that we were not conscious of at the time. We had a tribe mentality, we had self expression, emotion, a spirit that by its efforts grew because it was people-driven: tribe-driven, not herd-driven. Bolton Health Studio had heart, soul and leadership.

This concept, if that is the right description, would prevail for over thirty years. Throughout those years we would develop other things that attracted customers to our club in Bolton. One of those innovations was a self-development course of training to qualify people to work in the developing fitness industry. It would be this course that taught me, the 'tutor', to appreciate the power and the joy of the tribe.

Training people to work as a fitness instructor was a simple matter of teaching them the principle of exercise. To do this we had to teach them the techniques needed to deliver exercises like the standing press, the curl squat, rowing and pressing exercises. There were issues like correct breathing techniques and safety issues like lifting with the back, strength and other functional movements. All very simple things that are now standard procedures. What we discovered during that pioneering phase of our life and the development of our business had nothing to do with skill or technique, health, safety or the framework of exercise, but everything to do with leadership, inspiration and the soft skills of communication.

LEADERSHIP

In the thirty-odd years that we ran our business in Bolton, we came into close contact with over a hundred thousand people. Our success at pioneering the multi-purpose club attracted people from far and wide and when we launched our training and development courses that attraction doubled. It was not unusual to have a hundred people, mostly young, visit in the week, but keeping them interested and having them come back needed more than just showing them how to curl a barbell.

Teaching people the mechanics of exercise can be quite dull, so I and our team of presenters came up with a policy. We set ourselves a goal of sending the students away at the end of the course punching the air because we had motivated them.

This policy came about because we stumbled upon a teaching skill called Neuro-Linguistic Programming (NLP) which was relatively unknown in the 1970s but founders Richard Bander and John Grinder were to enjoy a huge success in later years. The personal development programme utilises many different skills, like rapport, mirroring, and using keywords in relation to the recipient's mode of learning. NLP activates certain parts of the brain to enhance a sharper mode of communication. Touch, visual and auditory skills are key to better relationships with other people. One day without being aware of what I was doing, I suddenly found myself motivating fifty or so students to get out of their seats to applaud a rather dull subject like the framework of exercise.

Roy Hawarden was a university lecturer and one of his subjects was psychology: it would be to Roy that I would turn when discussing this sudden response to my basic delivery.

'It's called Neuro-linguistics,' he said.

So off I went to buy the only book on the subject at the time called 'An Introduction to NLP'.

What I discovered that day by accident was an important element in what this book is all about. Communicating with our people is vitally important in developing the tribe instinct in those around us. Billy Leach, Ann Hunt and the teachers of The Fitness League all had that touch, that ability, that charisma: talking without words, non-verbal communication. By their words and actions they said more than a herd of a hundred million people can convey through propaganda, legislation or promises of a strange and more flexible Europe.

SOME CALL IT CHARISMA

On April 9th 1963, John F Kennedy honoured the British leader of World War 2. In his speech he referred to Churchill's skill of mobilising the English language and putting it to war. Both Churchill and Kennedy were great leaders and great orators. Their ability to motivate and inspire were made for their time. The radio was the vehicle of the day. Churchill's speech didn't mobilise just the English but millions upon millions to take up arms and defeat the evil in the world. Kennedy's speech of putting a man on the moon within a decade and returning him safely inspired two hundred and fifty million to believe in the moon project and in their country. Churchill and Kennedy encouraged Tribe behaviour, bringing forth a belief that we as human beings have the ability to enrich our lives, with the right thoughts, guidance and leadership.

We are human beings and we are different. We are Tribe.

One of the most outstanding examples of herd mentality was seen in Victor Frankl's book 'Man's Search for Meaning'. The story is of Frankl's survival of the Holocaust.

Under the rule of Adolf Hitler, the persecution and segregation of Jews was implemented in stages starting in 1933. Government legislation included economic boycotts and an exercise called the 'Night of Broken Glass', a programme aimed at systematically isolating Jews and finally exterminating them. Hitler's choice to spearhead this operation was Heinrich Himmler who would become one of the most feared men on the planet. Himmler was head of the entire Nazi police including the notorious Gestapo. He was the Minister of the Interior and the Commander of the Waffen SS and the home army. He was also in charge of the death camps in the east. Although Adolf Hitler held the ultimate responsibility of what became the Holocaust it was Himmler who planned the proposed extermination of the Jews.

Frankl's book is a story of survival; it is also a story of how belief and singular thinking separates the human race and the herd mentality from all the other species. Frankl found a way to live when millions around him were being shepherded into the gas chambers. We are all subject to false beliefs. People, regardless of race or creed, are through mass persuasion, steered to buy, agree, follow, or be led by others who take control, or lead us in another direction or course of action. The human mind, the brain, is made to adapt, to bend, be flexible, or shaped like plastic to reform or re-wire and it was Frankl who grasped this in his bid to survive.

Frankl found humour, he called it 'humorous light', a trick learned while mastering the art of living. He saw that the most trying thing can cause the greatest of joy; he found art out of suffering, hope out of despair. He was grateful for the smallest of mercies. The meager pleasures of camp life provided a kind of negative happiness. He even had a balance sheet of pleasure and pain and it would be the pleasures outnumbered by the painful ones that he found time to consider.

Victor Frankl had that rare quality that we often call leadership: he would be the one who saw hope when no-one else could. He would be the one who would laugh and bring humour to the ones around him when the others could only see sorrow. Frankl was a leader who had a heart and soul. Hitler had neither. Frankl ultimately destroyed Himmler because he was the source of this Tribe. Himmler only had his herd, who by definition had no guidance, no leadership, and no humour.

Frankl talks of being herded like sheep, of having a mind and looking for inner freedom, of descending to the level of animal life and feeling like one of that herd. Frankl defined the difference that makes the difference and that is the mentality that separates the tribe from the herd. He was also gifted with vision and that vision would be his saviour.

He had no news of his wife and family yet each day he would see them in his mind's eye. Frankl, like many others in this book, sees himself where he wants to be, not where he is now. He saw himself with his family and talking to his wife, little knowing that she, his mother, father and brother were all dead. But because of his vision, he saw them alive and sharing his conversations. His leadership and his vision set him aside from the people around him and because of that he gave hope to others. He had faith in his God and faith in himself and sufficient faith to take tasks on when all around him were avoiding the most arduous tasks like working with the sick. He would 'see' the events after the war and even knew how he could utilise the knowledge and skills that he learned in his years in the camps. His vision saw the formula for his work in Logotherapy, a therapeutic doctrine, a treatment for depression. Even when he was in the depths of despair, Frankl saw the future. His suffering became an opportunity to learn: he was surrounded by despair and acute depression and he later used those experiences to develop methods to help others after the war. Without vision and his ability to lead, none of what he did later in life would have been possible.

Frankl's philosophy was extremely simple and that was that he and he alone would experience the suffering, and only then could he really understand what other people were feeling. He believed that that was the primary reason for life. If life is worth living then that must be reason to exist. Purpose.

Leadership. The ability to see outside of one's existence and faith that there is a far greater force than ourselves.

I first read Frankl's book 'Man's Search for Meaning' over twenty years ago. As I write this book I am once again reminded of those qualities and I see those qualities in the people in this book. Billy Leach's simple way of life and the constant message that comes from Sylvia Faucitt's quote, that she looks for reasons to continue not excuses to quit; Derek Craynor's constant activity and non-stop life - 'to rest is to rust'; Doris, who at 90 is still going to her exercise classes; Lynn Ward and her mother of 94 and faith in The Fitness League; and John Higson whose commitment is to live to be a hundred. All show remarkable faith in their search for meaning.

The herd drifts or is shepherded in a certain direction and the masses follow. The leader of the herd dictates; the leaders of the tribes share. Leadership, vision, purpose and commitment are all qualities that are necessary in the ruling class.

ANIMAL FARM

George Orwell's 'Animal Farm' is a parable seen through the eyes of the child. It is a story of animals being the ruling class and the misuse of power. The story, thinly disguised, is of the Russian Revolution and how Stalin gained control, which would eventually lead to anarchy. In his book, Orwell used pigs as an example, leading the other animals and, when gaining power, finding it hard to resist temptation. Selfishness and hypocrisy lead to more and more power, and the disintegration of their society. All animals should be equal, but in his book he shows that, just like people, some are more equal than others. Leadership, like the Third Reich and Hitler's henchmen, has many parallels with Orwell's theory.

In Animal Farm he shows the ideals through the seven

commandments depicted through the Old Major, a rather naive mixture of Marx and Lenin.

His doctrine and 7 commandments are:

1) Whatever goes upon two legs is an enemy.

2) Whatever goes on four legs or has wings is a friend.

3) No animal shall wear clothes.

4) Four legs good, two legs bad.

5) No animals shall sleep in a bed with sheets.

6) No animals shall drink alcohol to excess.

7) All animals are equal but some more equal than others.

The fall of the Soviet Union in 1989 was a result that Orwell would have welcomed. His story told through the eyes of the child would become a text on the British curriculum.

9 – PURPOSE

MIRACLES AND THE FULL MONTY

He weighed in a little under ten stones and at five feet six inches he was muscular – not an ounce of fat on his wiry frame. It was midday and they had been hacking away at the coal face since six o'clock that morning. Their quota was six tons of coal and they had been at it for nearly six hours on a seam no more than four feet high. Backbreaking work: one man hacking away, the other shoveling onto the conveyor belt transporting coal to be loaded into tugs.

Working as a team they would change places every forty minutes, only stopping to drink a little water or eat their packed sandwiches. They were a thousand feet down and a mile from the pit shaft. A cage 10 feet by 10 feet; twenty others lowered into the darkness with only the light from their headlamps to guide them to their place of work. Six men would die that week in the mines across the country. Who's counting lives when there is a war being fought on the surface?

It was 8 May 1945 and the day that Winston Churchill announced that the war in Europe would end: VE Day.

The two men working side by side knew nothing of this. The six tons of coal was just another quota to be filled and with only eight hours to do it they dug away to fulfil their task. The news had not yet reached them that Adolf Hitler had committed suicide. They knew nothing of the celebrations going on above, only the sound of themselves and the belt that forever needed filling. That, and the creaking of the wooden props that held the million tons of rock, soil and coal above them.

Joe Heathcote and Jimmy Gregory shared a bond that can only exist in a world like this, where lives are continually at risk, conditions are extreme and the threat of injury or death is continually pushed to the back of the mind. Both these men were still young at thirty-four. One of them had a child on the way, a wife eight months gone, something to live for, work for, prepare for. All for the future after the war.

There is a well-practiced ritual when working down the mines. Necessary habits, protocol, systems, automatic processes and procedures, not unlike the troops above ground: habits to cope with fear. There are no habits, however, with Mother Nature. No warnings, just sudden impact, not even the snap of the wooden props, a lightning slap like swatting a fly and it's gone forever; a hundredth of a second in time.

It was Joe's turn to work the seam when it happened. But for the conveyor belt, Joe Heathcote would have been history as would Jimmy, his mate digging feverishly to drag him from the fifteen inch gap between the slab of rock and the conveyor. There would be more than one miracle that day. It was a million to one chance that the slab hadn't hit the belt; it was another miracle that Joe was still conscious. It would be another million to one that Joe would survive and yet another miracle that he would eventually walk again and celebrate the birth of his daughter Patricia.

I found out later in life that Jimmy Gregory carried Dad the full length of the journey to the surface, refusing all help from others. Jimmy Gregory and Joe Heathcote were members of a tribe, warriors whose battlefield was a thousand feet below ground. They asked no favours and gave none. When I asked Dad in the final few years of his life, what his favourite job was, he simply said 'The pit'. When I asked him why, he said just as simply, 'The camaraderie'. He would never work below ground again and when the world was celebrating an end to a global war, Joe Heathcote started his-war to survive his next sixty three years of life: for that he needed purpose.

The first thing Wynn Barber did when leaving the army in 1945 was to join the Women's League of Health and Beauty. Hamish McPherson on the death of his wife joined our gym in Bolton. Tony Ford, like Hamish, would find a purpose and a reason to live by joining his local bowling club after bereavement. Tony was seventy-eight years old then and now at eighty-four he is passionate about his pastime. All three of these people engaged their minds first by joining a group of people; secondly, they occupied their minds by buying into a pastime and therefore becoming a member of the tribe; and thirdly, they kickstarted the rest of their existence by finding a purpose out of despair.

FINDING A REASON: PART 1

I love the film The Full Monty and have watched it perhaps ten or twelve times. The film starring Robert Carlyle, Mark Addy and Tom Wilkinson, resonated with me, possibly because of my working class background. The film is about a group of guys who are on the wrong side of the fence. Sheffield, once the centre of the Steel Industry, would lose its hold due to the economic downturn in the early seventies and the oil crisis in the Middle East. The story of the Full Monty is about triumph out of adversity; about our so called 'no hopers': people who have lost their livelihoods, their self respect and their ability to get out of the rut. In their desperation, the group of people, led by Robert Carlyle, are persuaded to take part in a hare-brained idea of making money by being male strippers. The 'one night only' meant that they would strip to the buff for that one single night. One of the songs in the film is 'Keep Your Hat On', leaving everything comes off except the hat.

The film, now a stage musical, is hugely funny and shows the small group of men working up the courage to do the one night only. It also demonstrates the pathos and the hopelessness when people who know nothing else except steel find themselves ill-equipped to survive in a changing world where they have no control over their destiny, leaving them with little reason to live.

The chorus of the song 'Keep Your Hat On' goes:
"You give me reason to live
You give me reason to live
You give me reason to live
You give me reason to live
"You give me reason to live
You give me reason to live"

These six lines in the song, sung by Tom Jones, encapsulated the reasons for the film. Out of desperation they found a purpose in life and by doing that they found a reason to live.

It is said that we are the sum total of our experiences. I often wonder what would have happened if I had not wandered into the ward where there were all those children with leukaemia and my subsequent fortieth birthday endurance tests. Now at eighty-one I am still raising money in the same way. Testing my resolve for Cancer Research, the event on my fortieth birthday of running forty miles, lifting forty thousand pounds in forty minutes, playing four people at squash and doing four hundred sit-ups started a chain of events that is still going over forty years on. The fortieth would manifest itself once again at fifty years of age when I repeated it all again, this time in units of fifty. I don't think I would be writing this book if I had not taken on those events that have now become the sum of my experiences.

Experiences shape our existence. We as human beings walk upright on to legs, we have a creative brain, we invent things; we are different than any other creature on earth. We are special because of that difference and if we do not use these gifts, then we become no more than the sum total of much less than our capabilities. We are by nature herd animals and if we fail to innovate then we stagnate. The safety of the herd breeds complacency which lies on a path leading to nowhere. Finding purpose is like finding another path and by finding another path we have another world at our feet.

CARPETS, CHROME AND CONIFERS

Sometimes we just have to sit down and think there are all kinds of names for this, lots of clichés like 'blue sky thinking', 'white hat thinking' or the classic one, 'thinking outside of the box'. Whatever it was, the thoughts came out of desperation and probably out of reading a lot of books and talking to a lot of people.

It was 1968 and we had decided to try and make a living out of our gym. This meant moving premises, finding bigger rooms and generally spending money that we didn't have.

We had an impossible situation. We wanted to convert a gym that was full of barbells and dumbbells and a single bench and a contraption called a Power Pack and pretty much nothing else. We had a room sixteen feet by fourteen feet; white-washed flagstone floors, two light bulbs, no changing facilities and no running water: not by any stretch of imagination a foundation for a commercial health club.

It would take four years to find the answer and another three years to find the secret. You see the answer was simple. Make everything look good. The floors were covered in carpets, we decorated the walls, made those not too attractive barbells shiny with chrome and put the finishing touches in place by spreading some plant life around, making a harsh environment cosy. We also expanded our floor space from about two hundred square feet to 10,000.

We did something that was so unique it hardly seemed true, but it was. We installed a beauty salon, a crèche, a restaurant and a squash court. In simple terms, we broke all the rules. No-one, but no-one, put these things in a gym! Add to that music and movement (later to be called aerobics), a sauna and steamroom and we had a product that was twenty years ahead of its time and what is more it worked. Bingo! We had found the answer.

Not quite.

We had found the answer but we had not yet discovered the secret. What we did find was that all of the auxiliary features of our gym (that we now called a studio) attracted the customers but what it didn't do was keep them. We had a wonderful product, we had wonderful staff and we had a wonderful approach to business, so why did we have a woeful habit of losing them? That's when I sat down to think.

People leave health clubs and gyms because it's hard work, because it requires dedication, discipline and stickability, so we had to find a reason other then the product to keep them. We had to develop more. Not equipment, not beauty salons or crèches, nor in those days saunas or movement to music. We had to develop the stickability and that had nothing to do with the perceived product and all to do with having fun.

FINDING THE REASON: PART 2

Tony Ford had never played bowls in his life until after his wife, Jean died. He had said to her over her last few days, 'Save a place for me love, I will not be far behind you'. That was eight years ago. 'I didn't take to bowls immediately,' he said to me. 'It wasn't like the game grabbed me. It didn't, but after some time I decided to join a bowling club and I met a lot of people, so I joined another club. I now play about eight times a week, but more important than that is the amount of people I know.'

Tony went on to say that he knew about three hundred people from different clubs. 'It might just be hello', he said. 'I know most of them by name.'

We were sat on a bench watching a game. There was a friendly atmosphere and quite a lot of conversation around us. A few were drinking tea, some wine or beer. Later they might have a sandwich or a piece of cake. The small community obviously enjoyed this regular occasion. It reminded me of what we had put into place at our club in the seventies: I called it emotional glue and it was this that they had in abundance that night. Tony Ford was essentially talking about the social interaction that we call Tribe and that is what we created all those years ago.

We realised that if we could not find the stickability factor, then we would never hold onto our members, so that quiet contemplation of, if you like, thinking out of the box, created a social network that had nothing to do with working at their fitness, losing or gaining weight, or running faster or longer. We created that emotional glue through a social calendar that involved all of our members.

We had trips. Trips abroad, trips to Ascot, ski trips to Aviemore in Scotland and ski trips to France. We took our members to the Canary Islands and we took them to Hollywood in Los Angeles. We organised house parties and even cabaret nights. We had charity balls at various venues. If there had been quiz nights we would have done those too. We had open days and asked members to bring friends and we had games, treasure hunts and entertained them with a glass of wine and lucky dips. The social calendar matched our variable facilities and gave hundreds of our customers other reasons to bond them to our business. We gave so many reasons to keep their memberships alive that it meant a longer life with us, and more purpose to their lives. We realised that people buy people and the socialising of those people bound them to us.

Hamish McPherson, Joe Heathcote, The Fitness League, Tony Ford, The Full Monty, and almost every single person in this book, found purpose in what they were doing, not by the activity that they were in engaged in but by the people around them. Purpose and Tribe are one and the same.

10 – CHOICE

WHAT'S IN A NAME?

Among the many hits of Johnny Cash, one song resonated with the inmates of California's San Quentin Prison: 'A Boy Named Sue'.

The lyrics tell the story of a young boy who grew up to be tough because everyone had a go at a male with a female name. Names create our identity. If you are a boy with a girl's name you could be more likely to be suspended from school than if you have a boy's name. In a study at the University of Florida, economics Professor David Figlio conducted a study over a period of four years. He found that boys with names more suitable to girls misbehaved more and were most likely to disrupt their peers.

Studies also reveal that names are important for getting jobs. Mary will be more successful than Gertrude, Joe more acceptable than Humphrey. One study found that women with masculine names like Leslie, Jan or Cameron tended to be more successful in legal careers. In 2011, LinkedIn analysed more than 100 million profiles to find out which names are more associated with CEO positions. The most common names for men were short names like Bob, Jack and Bruce. In the same study, LinkedIn found that female CEOs were most likely to use full names like Deborah, Cynthia and Carolyn.

Names for individuals are important, but so are names for companies. I love the story of Joe Foster who had a small shoe-making business in Mornington Road in Bolton. Joe made rugby shoes and soccer boots and what were called running pumps. The business was formed a little over a hundred years ago and it was in the 1960s that a change was coming.

Jo Foster's two sons, Joe and Jack, were about to step into their fathers 'shoes' and take charge of the business. The corner shop in Mornington Road was to become a major player in the manufacture of sports shoes with Joe and Jack in charge.

The business moved to Bury, a small town seven miles from their shop in Bolton. The location, however, was not the only thing to change because the name Fosters and Sons was to be made redundant for Joe and Jack.

The letter arriving on Monday morning at their new headquarters informed the two brothers that their own name was not sufficient. The Government's Department of Registration and Brands revealed that Fosters and Sons had been registered with another company. Jack and Joe needed another name for their newly formed running shoe company.

On Friday evening of the same week, Joe informed his staff of six people that they had to come up with another name.

'I want you to come back on Monday morning with ten suggestions for a name.'

He too went home that evening and put his thinking cap on so there were seventy names on the table for Monday. Joe had no idea what the new name would look like but by 10 pm that night the magical name shone like a beacon in the sky and a new global product was born.

Joe came up with his brainwave on the way home. He decided to make a detour to the centre of Bolton and buy a dictionary from W H Smiths. He found that he had a choice: there was Collins Dictionary, the University of Oxford Book of Reference and the Cambridge Dictionary but in the end he chose Webster's Book of Names and References.

That night Joe sat down to scroll his way through the book, painstakingly analysing every possible opportunity for the new company's name. About three quarters of the way through, when he was very tired and ready to settle for another shift on Saturday, he found his name. The new brand leapt out of the page. The eighteenth word beginning with rh must have come from the gods because the name of the African antelope that was known for its ability to scale the mountains and difficult terrain was the rhebok, a slightly built indigenous creature that mirrored all the advantages of his shoes. With just a little tweaking of the letters, Joe Foster created the brand of Reebok, which would later become one of the most powerful brands in the world.

DECISIONS, DECISIONS, DECISIONS

Our brain makes dozens of minor and major decisions every single second of our lives. It is estimated that we consciously and subconsciously make 35,000 choices each and every day, from the second we wake to the moment we fall asleep.

When should I get out of bed? Do I stay or go? When do I brush my teeth, change my clothes? What do I have to eat or drink? Do I use my left hand or right hand to open the door? What transport shall I use? Do I pause, react, respond? What about breakfast, lunch, dinner? What dress, what suit, what shirt? What to read or watch? Who do I acknowledge? Do I smile, grimace, glance, stare, Shrug or not? Do I count calories, carbs, fat, protein? How about vitamins, minerals, amino acids? Decaf or regular, milk or no milk, latte, americano, cappuccino, chocolate or plain? Is this honest or dishonest? Do I vote, work out, drink tea, go for a beer? How can I say that I had no choice?

When it comes down to it, it isn't the major choices we make in life, career, or marriage that count; it is the everyday minor decisions that make life work for us. These are the words of Shad Helmstetter Ph.D., who came up with the 100 most important choices in your life that help to create your destiny.

There is an uncanny resemblance to what Helmstetter reveals and what is in this book. Number one on his list is not about our jobs or our choice of partner, or our homes or what school our kids go to. His number one choice is who we spend most of our time with. In number fourth position out of his hundred, is what you eat most. In seventh place is your posture and in eleventh out of a hundred is how much you exercise. Helmstetter's list of a hundred includes just a fraction of all the choices we make, that estimated 35,000, but his are the few that shape our future.

SERENDIPITY

Every time we make a choice there is always the risk of it going wrong. Just recently I attended a book launch of the celebrated author, Michael Connelly. Mr Connelly writes books on crime and important to his success is a central character called Harry Bosch, a Los Angeles detective. Connelly's character has helped to sell millions of copies all over the world and he ranks as one of top writers on crime fiction and I for one am a great fan.

The seminar was conducted as a one to one interview; so questions flowed on what made Michael Connelly and Harry Bosch so successful. The words luck and serendipity came into the conversation no less than seven or eight times during the one hour interview and when both he was asked why he chose crime fiction, he replied, 'chance' first before he mentioned 'choice'. Being in the right place at the right time makes up about ninety-five per cent of success and as Yogi Berra, the world famous baseball coach and off-beat philosopher said:

'When you come to the fork in the road, take it!'

Who knows what happens after we have made that decision. I spent forty years in business and I had to make decisions every day of my life that influenced the lives of my staff who relied on us to pay for their groceries, clothes, holidays, and everything that they valued. Taking risks is part of business and just as Michael Connelly and Yogi Berra say: 'We are all subject to chance'.

Making a choice about our eating habits or what exercise we take or how we conduct our lives outside of the necessities of just surviving, is a choice of preference. I prefer to be active. I prefer to be in decent shape. I prefer to eat my food of choice. I cannot dictate my future; I can only try to control it. I can, like Mr Connelly and Mr Berra, rely on fate to do the rest. Serendipity, hope and choice and the rest are all in the lap of the gods.

Joe Foster's choice of name was a choice of genius. Choosing a brand name is incredibly difficult in these modern times. When David Lloyd, the health club chain, was sold, Whitbreads stated that they had bought just two things: the name and the future. They paid £200 million pounds for the privilege. The choice of Reebok for Joe's shoe company attracted an American company and the price was agreed, based on the current market value. What Joe didn't know or for that matter anyone else, was that the market would change just one year after he sold the business. The running boom and other influential things like the preference for casual wear, tracksuits, jeans, shirts worn over pants, shell suits and many other things saw an unexpected drift away from the formality of dress. The whole western world embraced 'casual' and part of that was the athletic shoe including the running shoe becoming a part of casual dress.

Joe Foster missed the boom by months. Serendipity had dictated Joe's future. One year later, Joe would have made ten, twenty, maybe thirty times more for his very exclusive name, the name of Reebok.

TAKE THE SHOT. TAKE THE SHOT. TAKE THE BLOODY SHOT!

I don't suppose James Bond would have had the success if our hero had been called Jimmy Joint. Ian Fleming chose the name to suit the image of the man. In the film 'Sky Fall', our hero is seen fighting on the roof of a train travelling at a hundred miles an hour. Why two grown-up men should choose to climb on a train to fight is not explained in the plot. Coming to Bond's rescue is Miss Moneypenny, played by Naomi Harris, and she is listening to Bond's boss M, played by Dame Judi Dench, who is shouting down the phone for Moneypenny to take out the villain. But Moneypenny is faced with too many choices. Shooting at a moving target presents a harder choice than a stationary target, two men moving and fighting adds to the difficulty of choosing when and where. The mind is confused because Moneypenny has to think, act, decide and listen in s split second, and further to that decision is the fact that she knows Bond and is secretly in love with him. Forced into making that choice she pulls the trigger and Bond, played by Daniel Craig, is shot and falls off the train into the water below.

The opening words of the film; 'Take the shot. Take the Shot. Take the bloody shot!' epitomise the difficulty of choosing in the most difficult situation possible. Choosing our activity, our eating habits and our tribe shouldn't be too hard. Or are these actually difficult choices?

COMFORT ZONES

'I want you to teach him how to jump', said Frank Fletcher. Frank was referring to his son Paul, who had just joined Bolton Wanderers Football Club as an apprentice. Paul was just sixteen years old.

Paul had started his career playing on the right wing. It was at the age of 15 that he was selected to have a trial for England Schoolboys, and it was on this day that he noticed a young lad called Dave Lewis who played on the opposite wing. Dave was just 5'3" tall but when he jumped he would soar above his fellow players.

'He would hang in the air,' said Paul, 'and head the ball goalwards. It was uncanny: he wouldn't just do it once; he would do it time after time. It really was quite amazing. I was never called upon as a winger to head the ball, but after seeing Dave I decided to remedy the situation.'

For Paul Fletcher this was a moment in time. He went home and spent hours practising how to jump. He would go in the back garden of the family council house and practise heading the clothes line. It was at this point that became aware of Nat Lofthouse, the Bolton legend, who still holds the record for scoring goals for England on appearances (thirty-four goals in thirty-three games). He became aware of Wyn 'The Leap' Davies, another goal-scoring legend, and Tommy Lawton. All three inspired Paul and the inspiration meant that he changed to being a striker which was the start of an illustrious seventeen years at top level.

Paul's career was paralleled with the courtship and eventual marriage to Sian Roocroft. He tells the story when they first met at the Beachcomber Night Club in Bolton. He describes it as one of his greatest joys of his life, and I can vouch for that as I have known both Paul and Sian for nearly fifty years. There were many occasions when both of them would baby-sit for Brenda and me, watching over our two children, Paul and Karen.

Paul and I have been friends since his Dad brought him to me to help him to jump higher. Something I can take no credit for. I can take no credit for his choice of position or his choice of bride and I can take no credit for the next choice in Paul's life; and that was to choose his direction after the broken leg that halted his career in football.

Perhaps, just perhaps, I can take some credit for setting examples of what it is like to be aware of one's fitness. Perhaps this is why he had no hesitation in telling Nat Lofthouse of the gym where he had been training. Paul's recommendation to Nat, who was the manager at BWFC, resulted in the latter sending all the youth team to me for weight-training. Jim Conway, the youth team coach, brought some wonderful players to me and that started a relationship with players that still exists today. Among those to visit us over the years were world class players like Roger Hunt, Frank Worthington, Peter Reid and other big names in football like Gordon Taylor, now Chief Executive of the Professional Players Association, Nat Lofthouse, and later managers like Jimmy Armfield, Phil Neal, John McGovern and hundreds of other players, many who played at the highest level: Sam Allardyce and his wife Lynne, and the older generation, like Tommy Banks, Roy Hartle, Frances Lee and Rodney Marsh. All these and so many, many more forged a bond that still exists today. I knew so many players who had brilliant careers and who all helped to add richness to our lives.

This is perhaps why I understand how difficult it is for some players to see careers come to an end so early in their lives. Tommy Banks played for England with his brother Ralph, Nat Lofthouse died only a few years ago, as did Ralph Hartle, all of them players who entertained and brought pride and joy to millions of people, colourful characters who provided moments of magic for the adoring fans. It really is tough when it all comes to an end when you're just thirty years of age.

Paul Fletcher was just thirty when he broke his leg playing for Blackpool Football Club. Like many of his colleagues he had no idea what he was going to do. One minute you have a career and one tackle later it all comes to an end. Paul Fletcher had few choices. In his book he says: 'I had no plumbing experience, no joinery, I couldn't lay bricks, no office experience and I had nowhere to go'. Paul says that he made one more choice that changed his life, but I know that it wasn't one but four choices that changed Paul's life forever.

HOW TO WIN FRIENDS AND INFLUENCE PEOPLE

The first of Paul's choices was to concentrate on being a striker and his second was to go courting with Sian. His third choice was to enrol on the Dale Carnegie course in his home town of Bolton.

The Dale Carnegie course 'Install Confidence', teaches people how to speak in front of an audience and inspires people to look beyond their comfort zones. The fourteen-week part-time course tests you, forces you to stretch yourself and think on your feet. I did the course forty-four years ago and not once did I feel remotely comfortable with what I was being asked to do, but unequivocally it builds new horizons.

Paul called it 'Goodbye Comfort Zones'. He tells the story of just one two- minute spell in the thirty-two hours of the course. It was Brendan Fitzmaurice who drew a circle on the flip chart and inside the circle he wrote the word 'COMFORT'.

Then he asked the question: 'Where do you think you are going to make the most progress in life, inside the circle or outside the circle?'

The whole session lasts over an hour on the course but it is the blinding flash of the obvious that either strikes home or is lost in translation. For Paul, it was the moment of truth and that changed his life.

That choice opened the doors to a whole new career. He went on to build four stadiums: the McAlpine Stadium in Rochdale, the Reebok Stadium in Bolton; he was responsible for the stadium at Coventry and he worked on the new Wembley Stadium. In addition to that, Paul has consulted on thirty other stadiums across the world. He's been an after dinner speaker for over twenty-five years, speaking at football clubs, golf clubs, hotels, conference centres, world cup events, European championships and charity functions. He has spoken in Australia, Germany, France, Iceland, India and South Africa. He is an after-dinner speaker, a keynote speaker and a motivational speaker. He has met with kings and queens, presidents, prime ministers, rock stars, athletes and medal winners from just about every sport you can think of. his fourth choice was of course, to embark upon a new career.

11 – ACTIVITY

THE CREEPING RIGOR MORTIS

It is now sixty years since I came out of the army weighing 158 lbs. Now at eighty-one years of age I still weigh 158 lbs. The difference is that it is now in a different place than it was. The medical term for muscle wastage is sarcopenia and all of us will experience the condition. Muscle wastage starts in our thirties and it is hardly noticeable. The estimated calculation is about 3% per ten years. With regular exercise this would hardly show. By the time we are fifty, sarcopenia accelerates and certain parts of the body are more susceptible than others. The upper part of our chest, for example, the pecs, are the first to show the deterioration and for women it may mean a better bra is needed. The back of the arm, the triceps muscles also show muscle tone and muscle loss. The gluteus, the buttocks, start to sag and the quads, the frontal thigh muscle, start to lose shape and size.

Sarcopenia is nature's way of telling us that this precious thing called life will not go on forever and that if we have any sense then we should try to do something about it. The loss of muscle and the steady increase of body fat are generally the first signs of 'creeping rigor mortis'. The old saying that every day in every way I will get better and better applies to most things but not to getting older.

So what can we do about our loss of muscle?

Well a lot actually. One is that we can exercise, and two, we can exercise specifically. Exercise generally improves muscle tone and even muscle mass, but exercising with weights can be very specific so areas that suffer most can be accommodated specifically (see chapter on weight training). The ageing process can not be halted but we can slow it down well into our seventies, eighties and even into our nineties. Activity is good but specific exercise is better.

Just as exercise is important, so is the food we eat. Foods rich in protein such as chicken, meat of all kinds, fish, eggs, milk and cheese are all foods that will help to ward off sarcopenia. So will the breakfast cereals: muesli, porridge, shredded wheat. We can only cope with approximately twenty grams of protein at a time. A bowl of porridge with some milk will give you most of the twenty grams. Anything more than what the body can assimilate will be either passed away or stored and converted into fat. Good nutrition and a good programme of exercise is as near as you can get to staying active and looking good into old age.

It really doesn't end there. Sensible exercise and sensible eating will also nourish the brain. The connection between mind and body goes much deeper than just working out and eating proper food. Just being positive and thinking about what you do helps to create new pathways in the brain. Mary McDaid, Derek Craynor, Billy Leach, Sylvia Fawcett and so many of the people in our case studies are examples of a well-balanced way of life that may go on and on. John Higson's 'I will live to be a hundred' keeps John focused, positive and physically active into his later years and so it will with you.

'We should all be concerned about our future because that is where we will spend the rest of our lives.' Those were the words of Charles F Kettering, an American addressing the British Chamber of Commerce in 1989. Kettering was speaking the future of oil and business but he could easily have been talking about us and our health. Our future is really in our own hands and much of it depends on how active we are, how we choose our food, how we think and how we choose our Tribe.

Keeping going is not just the prerogative of the ageing population; it is for everyone who wants to keep active throughout life. Things start long before we even start to become old. Sarcopenia is just another word for muscle waste: exercise and sensible food will help with that but it will also help with our lungs, heart, our mobility, our balance, posture, the strength of our bones and our mind and the brain's ability to cope better when getting older.

Each of us is different: some people will see changes earlier, some later. When former World Boxing Champion Willie Pep retired, he was asked what went first.

'Is it your speed?' asked the reporter, 'Or is it your strength, or is it your timing?

'No,' said Willie, 'the first thing that goes is your money, then it's your timing.'

Well only a few of us are boxers but we can all be fighters when it comes to growing older better.

Charles F Kettering was right, we should be concerned about our future, we should demonstrate that concern by following the simple rules in this book and if not this book then just the people in the case studies. The real beauty is that we do have choices; there are dozens, if not hundreds of opinions. Just do something, make a start, get the body and the mind into gear and drive yourself into your future.

CYCLING, WALKING AND LOVE

Bertha Berry lived until she was ninety-eight years old. She should have died from scarlet fever when there was no known cure, but at three years of age she survived. Her parents, Mary and John Griffen, had to let nature take its course. Bertha, one of ten siblings, not only survived the killer disease without medicine, but grew up to cycle to work at the age of fourteen, a thirty mile round trip that she did daily, on the back of a ten-hour day in the cotton mill.

Without being aware of it, Bertha Berry had discovered that exercise and staying active would give her a long life, even against all the odds. Bertha continued cycling well into her twenties when she met and married William Berry, a miner. The twelve years of riding her bike ended when she found work locally. Bill and Bertha lived together until her husband died of a brain haemorrhage due to failing downstairs at home. From that time on she walked every single day of her life. She walked to work, she walked to the shops and she walked to church.

Bertha's habit of walking continued throughout her difficult life. Widowed at fifty and redundant from the failing cotton industry, she continued walking even when injured. You see Bertha Berry was accident prone; she broke her wrist falling in the street, and she broke her pelvis at seventy falling off the sink whilst fixing the kitchen blinds. Bertha had no less than eleven accidents, all at home or in the street and not once did she stop walking. Even after her broken pelvis she walked up and down the ward with a zimmer. She, like Sylvia Fawcett, never looked for the excuse; she always looked for a reason to continue.

Bertha Berry never did a day's exercise in her life. She only took medication when necessary and always stopped using it when seeing the first signs of recovery. She never showed signs of depression, probably because she always kept herself active. She never drove a car, boarded an aeroplane and only once did she travel abroad to Bruges. My Auntie Bertha live a very simple and yes, frugal life.

I spent some time with her on the day she died. She has just spent twelve months in a home and consistent with her life, she had walked from her bedroom to the communal lounge.

It was 11 a.m. and she greeted me from a chair with a beaming smile. I don't know to this day whether she had sensed something, a premonition, but she cupped her hands around my face and her whole body shook with joy. No words. No hello. No goodbye.

Late that night, Bertha Berry passed away. She was just a few months away from her ninety-ninth birthday. She said many times in the final few years of her life that she wished the good Lord would take her and that day he did.

Cycling and walking was all that Bertha Berry did but if there is a message here it is that by keeping active, having a loving disposition and finding her tribe with the church, she had found the answer to her eternal youth.

FINDING YOUR ANSWER TO ETERNAL YOUTH

The key to staying active longer is finding something you enjoy. It was Oscar Wilde who said that every time he thought of exercise he went for a lie down. So if that is what you want, then that is what you do. For the rest of us we need to find something other than satisfying our appetite for self-expression. Oscar Wilde was a man who had an immensely active mind and was exemplar of creativity. Sadly he died at just forty- six years of age.

Creativity is not just the prerogative of the literary world. Finding ways to help us live longer and better is left to others like the fabled Milo of Croton. Milo, a young farmer's son, always dreamed of being a strong man, but two thousand years ago there were no gyms, health clubs or even books to tell him how. The legend goes that Milo was watching a cow give birth to a calf and his Dad asked his son to carry the calf to another part of the field. Milo dutifully picked up the calf and carried it away from the mother. It was then that Milo came up with his idea. He would pick the calf up each day, and every day, and each and every day he would walk around the field and as the calf became heavier Milo would become strong. Greek Mythology does have a habit of exaggerating the truth, but most of us who believe the story of the young man from Croton who discovered the method that all bodybuilders and weightlifters abide by.

THE GYM

Two thousand years on from what started with a cow and a calf and a field, we now have health club chains, independent gyms and people all over the world pumping iron. What was once a myth is now a reality. Weight training has really come of age and fifty billion people all over the world have taken a membership to work out in the many different guises.

Today we can participate in a multitude of exercise classes from aerobics, pump, spin, yoga, palates, circuit, 24, body attack, step, high intensity, water aerobics, cross fit, and so many concoctions of the same themes.

Only a few of these classes demonstrate the principles of progressive resistance and none in the confines of the modern-day health club chain.

In contrast to 'the exercise class', the free weight areas are the only place where we can come close to the principles of progressive resistance. Still, the gym is with us and with that the opportunity to find the ideal way that will give you the chance to live a more active existence. Gym or no gym: unlike Milo of Croton, you do have a choice and here is what you now have.

WEIGHTS

It is now sixty-seven years since I walked into my first gym. The old King's Hall provided a choice of gymnastics or weightlifting and that was it. Today we have so much but let us start with weight training.

STRENGTH TRAINING

Weight training provides us with a choice of two alternatives: one is free weights and the second is the single station machines. Free weights, mainly barbells and dumbbells, develop better tendon strength, connective tissue and particularly the stabilising muscles that provide us with better balance.

If we look at Derek Craynor's programme, we will see that he uses a mixture of both. Derek's combination fits with studies across the world. Tufts University in Medford, Massachusetts has been pioneering strength training for older adults for over thirty years and Craynor's approach to weights at eighty-eight would support all the study's evidence.

Strength training benefits include reducing many of the symptoms associated with old age. These include:

Arthritis

Diabetes

Osteoporosis

Obesity

Back pain

Depression

Other claims include restoration of balance and a reduction of falls. This included a study in New Zealand with women of eighty and over who experienced a 40% reduction in accidents due to falling.

Studies at Tufts also show results in an improvement in

increased strength of bone mass and density. There is also a marked increase in muscle tone, size and definition. Very often there is a reversal of sarcopenia.

Weights also provide us with the opportunity to specifically target the problem areas like upper chest and the back of the arms, triceps and lower back in particular. This is to strengthen the posture muscles. This area is of particular interest to older people because we all 'shrink' with age. The large gluteus (bottom) is a particular problem with age: once again weight training can show significant improvement in this area.

There are very few other forms of exercise that can target these age-related problems. Aerobic exercises like running, swimming, cycling and rowing or the steppers, cross trainers, will give us the level of fitness but with weights we can be much more specific.

People like Hamish McPherson, Derek Craynor, Sylvia Fawcett and myself have all benefited from using weights. Weight training, weightlifting and bodybuilding did not just give me a level of fitness but provided me with friendship, community and for over forty years a livelihood. Who can deny good health, wealth and companionship, all from some barbells and dumbbells?

SWIMMING

Swimming is one of the best exercises we can do when we are in our advancing years. Dad taught me to swim when I was eight or nine years old. Now, 75 years later, I am still lapping the pool five to six days a week. Not only am I enjoying the benefits of swimming but I am still discovering new ventures, new challenges and even new ways that I can continue with the precious gift that Dad gave me all those years ago.

So why swim?

Well, a study by Bucknell University, Lewisburg Pennsylvania, claims that exercise is better in the water than out of the water with buoyancy being one of the great advantages. Bucknell examined the principle of swimming and said that statistically we have so many of the benefits because there is a continued overall resistance of more than 13% compared to exercising on land. Water aerobics, walking and swimming, all provide an excellent w: working out in the water means just that. We still have to exert energy to reap the rewards. Swimming will only work if you work at the swimming.

Fitness however is only one of the benefits. Swimming will help in combating the ageing process and the therapeutic benefits are great when recovering from accidents and sickness. Then there is social involvement, and I can verify that I have met many people In would not have met, had I not taken up swimming. I now have a whole new trine through open water swimming, pool swimming and a fabulous new experience. Swimming in Lake Windermere on the Great North Swim gave me more than swimming in open water. It gave me a challenge and an opportunity to open a whole new life at eighty years of age.

Other benefits of swimming are stress reduction and fun. Open water swimming can be contagious and to take part in an event with ten thousand others is just remarkable.

Flexibility, strength, endurance, more pliability with our muscle suppleness, balance and an increased cardiovascular capacity are just a few outcomes including weight control. The benefits go on. Here are some of them.

WATER WALKING

We can move forwards, backwards and sideways. We can take

long steps, short steps, quick steps, slow steps. We can even vary that in shallow water or deeper water.

WATER AEROBICS

Full body rhythmic exercises for 20 minutes provide cardio-vascular benefits. Doing all this can improve both upper and lower body, shoulder, chest, back, arms, upper legs, calf and even the core muscles through twisting and turning.

FLEXIBILITY

Large movements, full range lateral raises, i.e. arms going out to the side, to the front and to the back, work the deltoids (shoulders) and triceps and curling movements tone the biceps.

WATER RUNNING

Running in water is a great way to get our exercise. This was a rare sight in the past, now all kinds of athletes use water to both increase cardiovascular fitness without the impact of running on land. This is also a therapeutic strategy for rehabilitation.

Runners, cyclists, soccer and rugby players, all kinds of sporting activities can be done in water.

GET ON YOUR BIKE

The Tour de France is one of the greatest sporting events in the world. The fitness level of these athletes is a sight to behold. Cycling, however, goes way beyond the super athletes. It is a sport for all and a pastime I enjoy. It is also a quite wonderful way to get and stay fit.

Whether you are cycling to work, to school, going to the

shops or just doing it for the fun, the bike is without doubt one of the best exercises ever. Here are a few tips when starting out:

Practice in a safe place.
Wear a helmet.
Be seen and heard.
Check you bike.
Be alert and plan your route.
Don't forget the Highway Code.

HEALTH BENEFITS

Cycling is a great exercise to prevent heart disease. It is also great at fighting obesity and diabetes. To get the best out of you and your bike you need an hour to an hour and a half of steady biking per week. As you become fitter increase your time to about two and a half hours per week.

This will give you a stronger heart, a fit body and a healthy mind.

Cycling is also great therapy and a fine way to relax.

SENIOR CYCLING

Join a club. There are many who have regular meetings, park rides and there are clubs just for the elders.
Cycling gives us all the benefits that running, walking and swimming do.

The alternative to outdoor cycling is to use the indoor ones in your local gym or leisure centre. These won't help your balance or expose you to fresh air, but they are great for raising your fitness levels.

If you are using a gym then it might help if you combine cycling with some weights: free weights or machines. The benefits of using a bike indoors or out are almost limitless.

The gym will also provide a source of community (tribe). Talk to people, develop relationships, and follow the advice in the chapter on Tribe. The benefits increase immeasurably when you mix with people. Studies have shown and continue to show that it is not just about food or exercise, but about people and that means Tribe.

RAMBLING

The ever-growing popularity of walking is a testament to its value. Besides the fresh air, improved circulation and weight loss, walking is also low impact and that means that there is less stress on joints. For many walking is the perfect answer when getting old. Like all exercise it is good for the heart and therefore the cardiovascular system.

This gentle form of exercise is relaxing and especially when done on groups. It is well tested and it has been proven that is also affects the brain. All this helps us to sleep better and therefore makes for a more relaxed life.

Unlike the more robust pastimes, walking can be adapted to suit all people at the same time. Family, friends and mixed groups call all walk together.

There are hundreds of clubs throughout the UK and thousands across the world. In the national magazine 'Psychologies', Julia Bradbury, the television presenter, is considered to be the modern face of walking. Her passion for walking began when she was just six years old, walking the Peak District. I personally can't think of any exercise that could be better than walking in this extraordinary countryside.

Bradbury's television series 'Wainwright's Walks' and 'Railway Walks' have helped to inspire millions.

A rambler's survey revealed that 77% of UK adults, about 38 million people, walk for pleasure once per month. Of these

62% cover more than two miles at a time. Great stuff for the mind, body and soul.

Walking is great for clearing your head and as Fredrich Nietzsche once said, "All truly great thoughts are conceived while walking". Problems, puzzles and perceived issues of the mind can all be solved with a simple uncomplicated period of time spent just putting one foot in front of the other. Try it!

THE EXERCISE CLASS

I have yet to see anything better for older adults than The Fitness League, but with only twenty per cent of men taking part in group classes The Fitness League fall just a little short of perfect.

The health club chains live and die on their classes. It is now quite normal to see a hundred classes a week on any one single site. The fitness industry has embraced the exercise to music principle ever since aerobics came on the scene in the late seventies. We have a wonderful choice: zumba, pump, and spin 24, an intensely active class that lasts twenty-four minutes. There are yoga classes, pilates, circuit, boxercise and so many more. Ironically, the classes only appeal to women. Most classes, including the ones where they use boxing gloves, will only attract about twenty per cent men and sometimes not even that.

In the early eighties we made classes aimed at the men. We called then Fitness and Fatigues. They were very basic and were probably the early classes that we now call 'Boot Camps'. We even recorded them and put them on audio tape. The success was huge but they still only attracted about thirty per cent men. The psychology of group exercise unfortunately appeals mostly to the girls.

Any form of exercise needs something more than just

physical involvement if we are to get the best out of ourselves. Classes are great, but what they don't do is provide an end product. Yes, we can feel spent on completion of the class, but if we don't have something that will show results, i.e. weight loss or a positive change in appearance, then our mind will continually look for something more. The class is the short term fix and once over we start to think, what next?

Make no mistake, classes do fill a need and they allow us to express ourselves through exercise. They give us a sense of accomplishment by exerting energy. When we do this, the brain releases hormones like dopamine. This is often called the pleasure molecule because it is involved with reward. The brain contains something like one quadrillion synapses and produces about one hundred different neurotransmitters all of which come into force when we work hard in a class. Hard, honest work provides us with pleasure and that is why the exercise class is so popular. Another reason is because we do it together (Tribe). A well coordinated series of exercises, a feeling of triumph, an adrenalin rush of euphoria, not unlike a team effort when winning a game on the field of play in sport. Once over however, the feeling soon goes and the sense of achievement is gone.

Finding something that absorbs the mind and produces long term benefits like weight loss or reaching a goal or a better measured performance will have a lasting effect on your mind. The exercise class is the raging fire that burns itself out. The achievement of goals is a much slower burn and some-times goes on for ever.

One exception to this is the Fitness League. During my research, I was continually reminded of the League's history and how their classes developed friendships. The word laughter was said over and over again; and when I thought about friendship and laughter I came to the conclusion that one was about 'life' and the other about 'now' and there is nothing wrong with either and a lot right with both.

TENNIS, GOLF, BOWLS

People don't play tennis to get fit: they get fit because they play tennis. The same could be said of golf and bowls.

All three of these sports or pastimes are excellent ways to stay in shape. All three of these wonderfully absorbing activities are also wonderful ways of socialising. There is nothing wrong with socialising because it says so in this book. 'The problem is not the problem, but what the solution creates,' said Ted Levitt in his book 'Thinking About Management' and the problem with tennis, golf and bowls is that the secondary benefit of socialising exceeds the real benefit of these activities.

Golf, tennis and bowls will give you all the exercise you need and equally all the socialising you need. All three involve eye to hand coordination. All three engage the brain, the body and all three have a competitive element that does wonders for our feel-good factor. There is not perfect answer to growing older and remaining active to the end. Tennis, golf and bowls are great examples of enjoying exercise without it being the primary objective; a bit like the Fitness League. The ideal solution, if there is such a thing, is to combine the pastime with something that provides a little more, say weights or riding a bike or swimming.

All of these activities absorb the mind, with none of them perfect in isolation. Science and medicine are only just getting to grips with things like neuroplasticity and for that matter, sarcopenia. Both of these subjects and many more will help us to address the issues surrounding age and the growth of mankind. The population of the world is now three times greater than it was in 1940. Clearly we need to know how to stay fit and healthy. The cost of keeping the world alive will put huge demands on governments. Drugs and medicine are not the answer. Better health, more active minds are, and limbs capable of mobilising our body until it is time to meet our ultimate destiny.

THE PSYCHOLOGY

In the early 1980s I was privileged to be involved with some quite remarkable athletes. Our club, Bolton Health Studio, had for over ten years been recognised as being the best of its kind in the country. When everyone else were still running gyms, we had expanded into other diverse facilities that had nothing to do with working out, training or pumping iron.

By the mid 1970s we had squash courts, restaurants, a crèche for the children, sauna and steam room, and a conference room that hosted speakers and provided a training room for staff. All this was not just innovative but revolutionary in what was to become the fitness business and even later the fitness industry. In our own little world we had become the centre of the universe.

Because of this, we attracted people from all parts of society. Show biz people would visit us when appearing in theatres. Cabaret was at its highest then and the stars of the day would be our guests. We had people like Frankie Vaughan, a top singer of his day; Frank Ifield, another singer, would come to see us; stars from Coronation Street; Les Dawson and rock groups playing at the local clubs. It was the sports stars however; who we welcomed most; soccer players, cricketers, and squash stars like Jonah Barrington, Jahangir Kahn, Bruce Brownlee and many more who ruled the squash courts at that time. We were also host to the world's top bodybuilders; members of a sport that effectively started the trend in keeping fit, looking good and building muscle.

My background had always been in weights and partly because of our reputation I was asked to judge physique competitions, local, national and international, and for close on twenty years I judged at the Mr Universe competition in London. Because of this we hosted the top flight body builders and because of our squash courts we attracted the world's best.

Bill Pearl and Jonah Barrington were two of the very best at their chosen sports. Jonah was six times world squash supremo. Bill won Mr Universe four times, was voted the best built man in the world, was Mr America and in his time an icon in bodybuilding. To have the privilege of knowing these two legends was colossal. To have then under the same roof and share their ideas was a chance in a lifetime.

Psychology in sport in the early eighties was almost unheard of, so to listen to their views on both their physique and mental approach to both training and competition was fascinating. What struck me at the time was how different they were. Jonah's sport was all about movement, intensity and lung-bursting periods of drawn-out rallies, then short bursts of speed. Bill, on the other hand, was about long term preparation: a slow steady build-up, little or no competition until the big day. Squash is dependent on regularity with series of events that allows the player to keep sharp until the day. Body building competition is more static, less involvement for long period of time. Squash is about opponents. Bodybuilders compete, with judges' opinions deciding the difference. The psychology of both is in the preparation, motivational techniques, consistency and peaking at the right time. One is about the slow burn, the other about intermittent levels. Both are about visualisation techniques, self-talk and feeding the brain with positives day in, day out. Both sports are dependent on how they combine the mental and the physical pressures to reach that peak.

I would discover that both individuals had exactly the same approach and that they had a level of understanding of the pressures that came with being at the top.

12 – CLUBS NEED TO GROW OLD

One of my local health clubs was conducting free health checks for their clients: blood pressure, weight and body mass index. We all know that these are three so-called health indicators and quite controversial ones as doctors and health experts find it hard to agree on what is what.

Two of these clients were telling me how much harm it was causing. One of them was a very fit sixty-three year old, slim, active and quite amazingly versatile in her approach to her fitness and lifestyle. She swims, teaches classes elsewhere, does yoga and looks the part: a shining example of ageing actively. In reality, she epitomises the ideal sixty-three year old. Both she and her friend were, to put it mildly, shocked that they were judged to be at risk, one with high blood pressure and the other by being obese.

Health clubs bundle their way through the day-to-day running of their clubs. Yes, the mechanics are there, the policies, procedures and management structures, but their ability to engage society and relate meaningfully to people is woeful. This is particularly evident with older people. The 'Health Test' was conducted by someone young enough to be the grandchildren of the two ladies who had received inadequate training on how to conduct the exam and her social skills particularly with older people were insultingly draconian.

Clubs have now become community-driven. They now have a roll-out product, a systematic reproducible set of digits that provides an attractive set of figures for portfolio development and equity sale. In other words, 'buy this because it works'. Plant and engineering without emotion.

But there is another side, a potential alternative that

both enhances the product and grows the emotional glue of personal development.

Clubs now are designed to accommodate the young. The present focus is High Intensity Interval Training (HIIT). Intensity and age are completely out of sync. They are like oil and water, very difficult to mix. Apart from yoga and pilates there is little else on offer for the older adult. There is nothing like the Fitness League, there is not even a suggestion of older adult classes or even older adult teachers, no meditation, no relaxation classes, no slow burn programmes, nothing that suggests that we get together for fun. All too imaginative for the systematic approach, for the product-driven mind of the carousel builders.

The retail and service industry is totally dependent on being imaginative, on creating ideas to excite the customers. Fashion is a great example: there is nothing that changes more than the customer's perception of how they look. Motor cars have changed little over the years except in the way that they are marketed or the enforced legislation in safety and economic efficiency. Food had never been sold on its nutritional value, but on how it tastes and how it looks. All these products and more are totally dependent on how they are perceived and particularly on how they are created. Fitness, on the other hand, is not driven by emotional attraction, but by the physicality of the product. The industry, like every other industry, will respond to current changes. In fashion, it is the cut of the cloth, the height of the hemline, or the psychology of colour. In cars, it's shape, space, comfort and image. In fitness, it's about the physical challenge, HIIT, cross-training, revs per minute, demanding and challenging workouts. We buy clothes and cars because they make us feel good; we like to be seen in them because they draw acclamation and even respect. We buy clothes and cars to satisfy our need to express ourselves physically, but not emotionally. All this is good for the customer who can accommodate hard physical exercise but it has nothing to do with the ageing population. They in other words fend for themselves.

The ageing population in the western world is the fastest growing part of our society. Governments, institutions and corporate developments have a duty to think seriously, morally and ethically about providing healthy lifestyles, activity, self-reliance, and above all independence. These qualities do not come easily. Apart from the individual's ability to move and function, they need to feel that they still have a place in society. It is one thing to be functional and another to feel that you are not dependent on others, but independent of others.

This is an issue not only for health clubs, but also for governments and neither of them are addressing it fully. Some would say not at all. That one single incident of incorrectly managing a sample test highlights the problems we have with individual care. A fitness instructor in mid-twenties assessing people in their mid-sixties with charts that are in all probability in need of updating, and the young man having no training in social or consultancy skills. This bodged-up version of a fitness and lifestyle assessment is an example of how casually the health club industry treats the serious implications of lifestyle. Health clubs are guilty of filling buildings with facilities, equipment and systems without the moral or physical support to back them up. This inhuman approach invites criticism, misuse of equipment, accident and emotional disturbance, with all of this contributing to the reasons why people leave. It is no secret that the industry performs badly in retaining customers with less than fifty per cent being average. The fitness industry has a huge opportunity to address the real issues of health and fitness into old age. It is unlikely to happen because there is no specific driving force in government and if it is to come about the person to head it would need to focus on bringing together the public and private sectors. The other essential is the knowledge needed to implement a health and fitness philosophy, the mantra that is evident in the characters in this book.

MOBILISING HEARTS AND MINDS

The Fitness Industry Association (FIA) was formed in the late 1980s. Prior to this, the industry had such a collection of moms' and pops' clubs or individuals who wanted to make a difference or pursue a dream to expand a hobby.

I was one of these stalwarts and with a few others formed the FIA. Our ambitions at that time were somewhat blurred: we knew that the 'emerging' industry needed managing, with controls that would set standards and effectively provide a mechanism to lead the cottage industry into the future, hopefully a future that would improve the health and fitness of a nation.

Somewhere on that journey paths would peter out, roads would lead to nowhere and the absence of funding would leave the FIA at a crossroads. Something needed to change and this change came with re-branding the FIA to UK Active.

Somewhere on the journey and the transformation, the rather hazy direction of the FIA was lost and with it went the secret to eternal youth. Strategies, vision and drive create change and the change needed now is to gather the information that we already have and mobilise the knowledge to reach the hearts and minds of government and private enterprise. Reform is not a word that we know in the industry of health and fitness, we only hear this when governments implement change, but these two sectors need to meet and if they do then great things will happen. The country is awash with money, much of it being spent on sickness. If that isn't on drugs and medicine then it is spent on the over-burdened National Health Service, a magnificent warrior of morality now spent and crippled with age and infirmity, much like the nation that it serves.

The nation under-exercises and stumbles along with little or no guidance on how to be active into old age. Clubs need to grow older with their customers, not just in facilities, but in structuring the requirements of older adults. These can no longer do any form of impact exercise, plyometrics, or short sharp bursts: age imposes a multitude of restrictions, both physically and mentally. The psychology dictates that we socialise more and exercise less: we want to be in the company of others not just in our age groups but a mixture of both. We still want our independence but we want respect and more than anything we want to exercise and communicate at the same level. Currently we are being served by staff who are often thirty, forty or even fifty years our junior. There is a different language, a different mentality and a different humour. None of this is addressed in training the young adults to converse with their elders. For everyone who is over thirty there are a thousand customers over fifty, not a huge gap to breach but many of that thousand are sixty, seventy and eighty year olds. Some clubs already make provisions and even offer 'free' memberships for the over-eighties, but they are few and far between.

When I asked about the two ladies, one with high blood pressure and the other with obesity, I wasn't met with an answer but with an accusation:

'We didn't say she was obese, he *(meaning the fitness instructor)*, would not say that!'

Without any provocation the enquirer (me) was called a

liar, when all I did was ask a question. An act of denial? A defensive answer? No... or just a casual confirmation with a customer?

All this reflects a lack of training in customer service, people skills and social interaction, none of which is contained in the specifications for a fitness instructor. Clubs provide facilities, policies and procedures, meet health and safety regulations, learn the latest techniques on teaching fitness or what to do if a customer has a heart attack, breaks a leg or faints in the sauna, but nothing on how to communicate.

If we are to improve the health and fitness of a nation into old age we first have to win their hearts and minds. If there is a system for checking the quality of the pool, then why not a system for checking the quality of instruction? There is always a policy in monitoring repair and renewals, profit and loss, but not for why people leave or cancel memberships. Investment in new technology, new innovative machines like treadmills or the new spin bike or the latest boot camp addition, franchised class or energy drink, flavoured water or high protein shake. All this encourages trade employment and customer interest but what are we doing about dementia.

EVOLUTION

How simple life would be if nothing ever changed. But it does. Forty years ago we set up our club in Bolton and I now witness that quite incredible progress. We have some wonderful clubs, spacious, well equipped, clean, organised, and a staggering amount of exercise options. Our industry is buoyant: there are something like forty billion people worldwide who have taken out memberships at the clubs similar to where I train in Bolton. The new budget club phenomenon just adds to the growth that I and my colleagues started nearly half a century ago. The dream came true but has now ended. We have woken up and what we now see is an entirely different product and whilst everything looks good on the surface, the industry needs to change. Technology changed all industry: cars are now almost perfect in design, flawless in engineering and quite incredible in their function. Television beams the stories as they happen; we watch world class tennis, golf, soccer, rugby and every manner of sport, politics, lifestyle and news at any given moment in any given day. The internet provides unlimited knowledge; our mobile phone gives instant access to everything and everything is available at a push of a button. The health club business however, is still the same with little or no innovation except the reinvention of the same. We had aerobics in the 70s, single station machines in the 80s, electric treadmills in the late 80s and early 90s and the exercise classes are simply a reinvention of the same wheel. With all the progress in science and medicine, and particularly neuroscience, we now know how the brain works and how we can enhance lives with the brain's ability to function through exercise. The whole world is applauding neuroplasticity (the flexible brain) and we are not even watching or listening or doing.

Brain training is exercising. Walking, running, jumping, lifting, exercising to music, swimming, in fact all kind of classes will exercise the brain, help and prevent the onset of dementia, help stroke victims recover brain traumas. In fact all kinds of disabilities can be cured in part and many times in full, yet the fitness industry still looks to reinvent circuit training and call it HIIT. The whole world is evolving and we just stay the same.

The FIA should have been around to implement the change. It is now UK Active. The FIA was to have had a political influence. Governments are desperate to reduce to reduce the crippling cost of illness. The arms are open wide to welcome a solution: investment is not the problem; leadership, courage and decisions are.

Wouldn't it be wonderful if the fitness industry was to be seen to have the maturity to take on the responsibility to enhance the lives of the people of this country, particularly those of us who are becoming old.

13 – ZONE

There is a lot of attention and publicity around the word 'Mindfulness' these days. Not a word that was part of our dialogue or conversation in the past but now, well, it's just part of the modern day culture. Defining the word is not easy but basically it means just focusing the mind on one thing and excluding everything else. The aim is simple. Just shut out the rubbish in life and cleanse the mind. It is like detoxing the body of impurities, another term we never talked about in the past. This time it is not about the mind but about the body and exorcising our digestive system of all impurities. Whether it is mind or body it's not a bad idea from time to time. Spring clean comes to mind or even an oil change after 20,000 miles in the car.

Focusing the mind is an essential of life. What we do to do this is a matter of choice. That said, 95% of the people I interviewed never engaged in detoxing. 90% only dipped into some form of meditation or mindfulness and no-one talked about fasting. To give any or all of these specialised areas some concentration needs more than just trying. What it does need is total commitment, determination and consistency. We now live in a world of so many conflicting ideas, theories, opinions and contradictory evidence that we are being dragged from one idea to the next.

Each week something new will be shown on television. Live longer by eating walnuts or juniper berries or drink the latest infusion of herb teas. Sugar right now is public enemy No. 1, closely followed by processed foods. Over the last decade or more we have been warned about alcohol. Beer and wine will give you cancer, Alzheimer's, dementia and anything else that is in the public domain at this moment in time. Health issues are great copy for newspapers, television, magazines and social media, none of which are studied in depth. All have conflicting evidence, all pull us one way then the other, all of these theories prevent us from really testing our resolve and in almost every case we are left not believing our own convictions.

'If you think you can, if you think you can't, you're right', said Henry Ford.

Henry Ford was talking about self-belief. He believed that the world would embrace the motor car and he proved that by making a million Ford Model Ts. An old colleague of my industry, Jack Lalanne, believed in hard exercise and fruit juice. Jack lived until he was ninety-five and was active till the end. Fruit juice is heavy in sugar even without sugar being added. Another person hailing from California was Fred Grace, a health nut and controversial character. Fred's articles in the Iron Man magazine had a host of followers including me. Fred Grace lived to be well into his nineties and was running till the end. Fred's diet consisted of a gruel-like porridge and he swore by a life of everything in moderation. When interviewing Derek Craynor, John Higson, Hamish McPherson and all the ladies of the Fitness League I saw a pattern that has nothing to do with their diet, exercise or anything that is the latest fad on television, or in newspapers, magazines or social media, but everything to do with their own values and beliefs gained over years of practice and a history of consistency. Each and every one of them has developed an ability to zone in on what they believe and somehow resist the constantly churned-out garbage that can grab the headlines.

Zone means now.

Being in the zone means living in the moment. Zone means meditation if meditation does it for you. Zone means yoga and it also means the run or the workout in the gym. Zone for me means my swim. Zone for me for over thirty years was my workout in the gym, then my zone changed to my running. My zone was also my family: Brenda, Paul, Karen and later my grandchildren Joe, Matthew, Sam and Georgia, and now my great-grandchild Sofia Rose and her mother Charlotte. My swim, my family, my work were and have always been my zone, my absorption in life. It is them, these things, this time, this day, this hour, this minute that is the zone. It is not me; it is what I do.

When I asked Derek Craynor if he had a mantra or philosophy, or a certain belief, he answered: 'My grandmother always said that to rest is to rust.' The seed that Derek's grandmother planted over sixty years ago grew into a belief which became a way of life. That way of life became Derek's zone and that is where he goes to provide his mind with his peace. Jack Lalanne, Fred Grace, Mary McDaid, Sylvia Faucitt and Ann Hunt know where to go to find their peace of mind: they go where we all go to find our zone.

Peace of mind comes at a high price in today's topsy-turvy world. Everyone wants to be part of the growing economy and to achieve that, people need to join the rat race. There are pressures to make more money and to spend more money, keeping pace with our peers at home, at work and in our social lives. Add pressure on pressure. Peer pressure in schools today is probably at its highest ever. The advancement of technology puts many of our younger people under even more pressure. Phones, social media, fashion and appearance all add pressure onto more pressure. The young, the middle-aged and our older generations each have their own world and to escape from these pressures we all need another world to escape to.

I remember giving a talk to a group of businessmen in the mid seventies. We had been in business ourselves for about four years and we were under a great deal of pressure to succeed.

This was a time when we were trying to keep pace with a massively growing industry. We had about two thousand members at our club in Bolton, with over five hundred attending each day. They were all being attended to on a personal growth basis. We were open from 6 am to 10 pm seven days a week. Within our complex we had a restaurant, a crèche, a beauty salon, squash courts and about half a dozen 24/7 amenities. I was involved with trying to become a national trade representative and the pressure from the customers and our staff were enormous. Add to that an athletic career and judging at events including the Mr Universe competition and other commitments such as fund-raising for charities, my commitment to family and a social life to boot. The group of businessmen I was speaking to knew this and asked how I handled it.

Tony Rink was the one who asked the question.

'How do you find the life balance?' To be quite frank and at that moment in front of a hundred successful people, I didn't know how to answer but out of nowhere the answer came.

I drew three circles on a flip chart. In one circle I wrote 'FAMILY', in another circle I wrote 'WORK' and in the third I wrote 'ME'.

In explaining what I meant, I said the family is the most important thing on earth, so in order that I can look after them I need to earn money to fund our lifestyle. To do that I have to work and my work was my club. Under each of the three circles I wrote six priorities; things like: holidays, standard of living, cars, schooling, clothes and trips. Under the circle on WORK I wrote: income, satisfaction, ambition, staff, income and expenditure and growth of the business. Under ME I put my training, my fitness, and my strength for without these I cannot look after my family, my staff or my customers.

Tony Rink, who asked the question, was a real mover and shaker in the community, an athlete and a very successful business leader. Without that question, I would never have put that basic life plan together. I had never thought that I even had a life plan, but obviously it was there all the time in my subconscious mind. The big lesson I learned from that exercise was how much better it is to write your thoughts down.

There is a huge advantage in changing the psychological to the physiological. Putting pen to paper registers something in our inner psyche that needs to be brought out into the open. Writing about it, talking about it and sharing it is one of the best lessons about life that I learned that day when Tony Rink asked that question.

Diaries, training logs, exercise programmes, repetitions and sets written down, recorded and there to be remembered; business plans, architects drawings and plans, the captain's log, a wish list and the six things to do today, the bucket lists, and the reminder list are all physical reminders and stimulators to get us going.

ISOLATION

Jim Halliday, my first weightlifting coach back in 1950, told me of his time spent in a Japanese prisoner of war camp in Burma. Two things kept him alive: keeping clean and finding that morsel of food that kept at bay starvation and death. Jim came home weighing just six stones and would go onto win the British Championship at middleweight within a year. He had the rare quality of shutting everything else out, except the one thing that occupied his mind. Weightlifting contains this rare opportunity: one single lift, one moment of concentration, just one isolated out of mind, out of body experience that is generated solely by the individual. There is no room for error: everything needs to flow. Weightlifters called this the 'groove', it was either there or it wasn't. Jim Halliday was gifted with a unique power. We know now that we have fibres in the muscle that are termed fast or slow. Twitch power among other things is generated by fast twitch fibres. The insertion of tendons into the bone and muscle dictates our ability to lift more by the leverage of these tendons. Long function influences that explosive power and the combination of all the above separates the explosivity from the slow twitch fibres, shorter levers of the tendons and the slower lung function of the distance runner.

Jim Halliday had all the necessary attributes and he also had the mind to use his god-given talents. He had the ability to zone in on exactly what he had set himself up to do. One of his party pieces was to jump onto a stage four feet high. He did this standing jump with his back to the stage. This needed acute concentration, a steady nerve, and courage and he needed to be in that part of the brain called the zone.

MEDITATION

To study, to ponder, to plan or think deeply and continuously reflect: the act of meditating involves deep reflection, especially on sacred matters. All deep thinking requires concentration and to do that we need to exclude thoughts that interfere with the object in hand. Mindfulness is a word that seems to grow in popularity when the world is troubled and when we have time to ponder our troubles. Mindfulness was never used during the Second World War. I never remember the word being used on the building sites where I worked. I spent over forty years working with people who wanted to improve their physical fitness, to slim, or increase their strength or physical ability. For many years I worked with disabled people, some of whom were athletes. In that forty year period they came and went; people of all ages, all sizes, young, old and across every range of ability, intelligence and willingness to commit or just go through the motions. Not once in those forty years did meditation become an issue or even a passing subject.

At first glance, we might think that mindfulness by definition means filling the mind but in fact means emptying the mind of the very things that fill it with the troubles of our time. It can be developed through the practice of meditation and the cult following of this mastering of the mind can be synonymous with prosperity. The Beatles never studied meditation until they became successful. The latest Hollywood stars when climbing the ladder were too busy climbing to meditate. Pressure in life creates tensions, neuroses and breakdowns, so we need to fill our minds with something that is productive and fulfilling. The Fitness League and almost all of the people in this book seem to fill their time with simplicity, friendship and enjoying what they do. Mental health is not for this book. I have interviewed some extremely competent people with years of experience. If there is a message to come out of this book and my experience it is that we need to listen to the likes of Sylvia Faucitt, Derek Craynor, John Higson, Mary McDaid, Billy Leach, Joe Heathcote and the thousands of women in their Fitness League.

I don't have any theories on meditation. I only know that for the past seventy years I have always tried to get absorbed in what I do. I didn't like the army: I was called up for National Service and conscripted into Her Majesty's Forces. After that I had to try and do what I had to do. At times I hated it, so you do what you have to do. Ironically, the lessons I learned did stand me in good stead later in life. I never thought that

I would go into business but on finding myself in a world of commerce I absorbed myself in a career that was so rich in knowledge, people, challenge and fulfilment that I had no time, inclination or even curiosity to fill my mind with anything else. The early days of weightlifting, bodybuilding and wrestling, getting married, having children, struggling to make ends meet, running, swimming, supporting charities, being involved and thinking of others left little or no time to seek out other things. My mind was too full with what I chose to do.

Weightlifting isn't as trendy as pilates, yoga, the latest trend of HIIT (high intensity interval training), mindfulness or meditation. Weightlifting, and especially Jim Halliday, taught me everything about concentration and zone. When we lift very heavy poundages there is nothing else that exists in this world except the weight and you. It is a moment that fills the mind to capacity. You may achieve this with yoga, pilates or even HIIT, a walk, a run, a bike ride, a game of bowls or whatever absorbs you. Perhaps even meditation.

OTHERS

Studies across the world are now revealing that what contributes most to activity in old age is not diet or exercise, but involvement with other people. These studies seem to support what I say in the chapter on Tribe, in particular the Fitness League. Certainly this comes out of my studies about the bowling clubs and the communal spirit. This is consistent with the six places in the world: Okinawa, Sardinia and places like Loma Linda in California. All these regions have a history of longevity via eating frugally and exercising, but mostly through lifestyle. The common denominator is not food or exercise, but community, thinking of others, taking action and being involved. This is covered in other parts of this book, but it is worth reiterating that nothing is more important in life then being a part of something bigger. Thinking about community may very well get us nearer to the zone than just thinking about ourselves.

14 – FOOD

The food of our lands in its natural state is the food of the nations and has sustained the planet since human life existed. Eaten in moderation with limited infusion of additives, processing and hygienically stored, our food will go on to provide life for mankind for as long as there is a mankind.

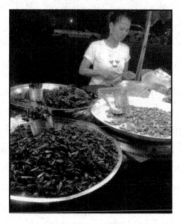

Street Food in Cambodia

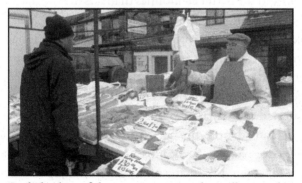

Paul Fletcher – fishmonger at a Lancashire village market

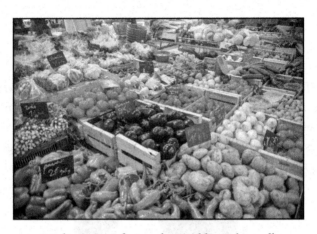

Mediterranean fruit and vegetable market stall

Branko Milanovic is a leading scholar on the subject of inequality, and is the author of the book 'The Haves And The Have Nots'. The book looks at some of the world's poorest economies and how they compare with more affluent societies around the world. One statement in the book, for example, was to show the difference between living standards in India and the United States. Some of the richest people in India, for example, are poorer than some of the poorest people in the United States. Food is more readily available in America, Britain and the better economies than it is in Somalia, Nigeria and Mali. Although food is not the subject of Milanovic's book it does in no uncertain terms spell out that inhabitants of wealthier countries indulge in food far more than those where food is a necessity rather than an indulgence.

For the first quarter of a century of my life I almost never questioned the availability of food. I do not remember having a refrigerator before the age of fifteen, I was at least thirty before I even heard of avocados and I never saw a real banana before I was ten. Like many of my generation, food was never a problem until you had none and for most of the war years food was rationed. Rationing went on after the Second World War up until 1950 and after that the situation improved but not necessarily from a nourishment point of view. In those early days, we ate to live. Now things have changed as we find more and more people living to eat.

Food is now fashionable. Food is now on a par with clothes, cars, homes, technological gadgets and baby shows. Food is a status symbol not just for the rich but for the poor as well if you live in the wealthier countries. There is a huge availability of the most exotic foods. Fruit and vegetables, fish and meat are all in abundance and nearly always well within the income levels of those who live in the more affluent countries, like Britain, America and the best placed countries of Europe. In terms of food availability we really never had it so good. So what's the downside?

There is a concept called Parkinson's Law. This by definition means that everything expands so as to fill the time available. Cyril Parkinson, a British historian first observed that government bureaucracy expanded as it became more efficient. We as a nation or nations have expanded our capacity for food as it has become more available and we have now become spoiled for choice. Our appreciation of its value is now less: we see food not as a nutrient but as an indulgence.

STREET FOOD

For anyone who has ever visited the town of Pompeii, you will see the ruins of a small street that used to sell just food. These were small outlets known as thermopolia, small restaurants that sold hot food that one could buy and eat without having to spend time being served. Eating out two thousand years ago. Eating out in those days was the predominant food activity for the poor. The thermopolium was the McDonalds of its day. The food was inexpensive, quick and filling. The fare of the day was baked cheese with honey i.e. protein, fat and carbohydrate. Pizza and spaghetti were also on the menu. Tables and seats made from wood were available and gambling could be one of the attractions along with a brothel upstairs for the more adventurous patrons. These street food vendors were the equivalent of the open markets that we have in towns across the world. Spain will have its tapas, and if you travel east to Cambodia, Vietnam and Thailand you will be served with frogs' legs, shallow-fried crickets, snake and tarantula spiders. France will serve you frogs' legs, snails, crepes and chips. Street food was originally conceived to satisfy the poor, only because the poor had no kitchens to cook in. Today that has now been reversed and eating out is for the rich and it is we who are now rich enough to eat out.

FOOD IS FOOD

The bottom line is that food is food. Anything that is available and is free from poison is food. No matter what eat, it nourishes our bodies and minds. Snake or tarantula, shallow-fried crickets and the street food of Pompeii will all give us protein, fat and carbohydrates. Here in the U.K., we will have shrimp, crab or prawn. Billy Leach in his day had minced meat wrapped in a cloth and boiled in a pan. Billy's cow heel pie, tripe and black 'pudden' is equivalent to the snakes of Cambodia. Pizza and spaghetti are the basic food of Italy. Tapas, the cheap food of Spain, has sustained the country for centuries. Indian food, Chinese and Japanese food are the food of the land, the sea, and the livestock of those countries. We are all living creatures of this planet and it is our planet that we turn to when we wish to live. Food is just food and it is only when we indulge that we turn to our nemesis and encounter the word diet.

Now after a full year of interview after interview, six decades of trial and error and soul-searching and sometimes hilarious experiments, I have come to the conclusion that the word 'diet' should be cast aside, eliminated from the dictionary and banned by the press. The word 'diet', by its own definition implies that it is something to go on, and by that suggestion it means that we are programmed to stop and come off it. It is a non- permanent fixture, a transient phenomenon, a temporary adjustment to our daily life, an excuse for mistakes of the past, an ideology, the yoyo syndrome, something I am going on tomorrow, when all that is needed is 'change'. Diet is the saviour of the press. Each and every day we are bombarded with the new way to slim, the diet that will change our lives, the new eating regime that lasts until the next new eating regime comes out. The easy, easy diet, the diet that eliminates hunger, the fat-free diet, the high fat diet, the high protein diet, the low carb diet, the everything that is white is shite diet, the chew it but don't swallow it diet, the six or is it eight meals a day diet, the five a day diet: page after page, week in week out, the weeklies, the books, the blogs, or anything by another name all write about diets. When all it takes is to eat less.

In the past twelve months, I have met with hundreds of people, spent an immeasurable time with dozens of therm and narrowed them down to fifty. Not one mentioned the Mediterranean diet. Not one mentioned the five a day: not one uttered the word diet. I saw only a few bottles of water. Fish and chips, lamb chops, fish and chicken sandwiches were mentioned in ninety percent of my interviews, as were porridge, Shredded Wheat and berries; meat and two veg, no meals between meals, only cups of tea and coffee. No mention of protein drinks, flavoured water or replacement supply. Not once was the word 'diet' used; they ate to live, not lived to eat.

EATING OUT

For quite a number of years I was involved in training staff to work in restaurants. Paul, our son, made his name by cooking some of the best food in the country. This earned him two Michelin Stars. For a short time I worked with some of his front of house staff on customer care and creating moments of magic for people who chose his Longridge restaurant to eat at. Top flight restaurants tend to select staff on their natural ability to serve: people who have good communication skills and are generally good with people. Such people are generally thin on the ground particularly when you are in the out of the way places in the North of England.

I evolved a mantra that said 'People don't eat out because they want to eat out. They eat out because they don't want to eat inn.'

Now there is a subtle difference here which takes us back to Pompeii. In those days the poor ate out only because they had no place to cook and they only bought cheap fast food. Today everyone has a kitchen and almost all of the time, cooks there. But in doing this, they tire of cooking so their rare forays into the world of eating out are a break from eating in. My words to front of house staff would be 'Make sure that you create enough magic to bring them back.' Customers rarely complain when they get decent food and decent service yet it doesn't surprise them that they don't get these enough of this. Food is food, service is service: just get these two things right. Food is food, so why should it disappoint if it's just food? Most of the answer to that lies not in the food but in our minds, as this next story will show.

THE £100,000 CUSTOMER

Mr Shepherd was a once a week customer at Paul's Longridge restaurant before he won his stars. One day Mr Shepherd, a teacher at a local college, came for lunch. He usually dined alone, but occasionally brought visitors to the restaurant to discuss business. One day he came in alone, just as he had often done since Paul had opened. This was a time when Paul did all of the cooking, so when the food went out he knew it was right.

The day after Paul received a letter from Mr Shepherd to say how disappointed he was with his meal. This mystified Paul, because he had sent the meal out, he had cooked it, and he knew that it left the kitchen perfectly presented and cooked to perfection. This was at a very testing time; Paul was trying to create a good reputation, but it was hard going in a small remote village near Preston.

That night Paul phoned and asked my advice.

'It was spot on,' he said, 'food and service was perfect.' So he was reluctant to pay for something that wasn't his fault.

'It only comes down to two things,' was my advice, 'you either value Mr Shepherd's support or you value your reputation more.'

Paul decided to reply to Mr Shepherd's complaint and offered him a free meal. Mr Shepherd continued to support Paul and even brought other people to increase his spending power.

Many years later, I asked Paul if Mr Shepherd still came into his restaurant.

'Yes,' he said.

We calculated that Mr Shepherd had been a customer for over twenty years. I asked Paul how much Mr Shepherd spent on a yearly basis. After a little thought Paul deduced that he had spent about five thousand pounds. Five thousand pounds for twenty years is a hundred thousand pounds. Not bad for relinquishing his pride for a day.

IT'S ALL IN THE MIND

Derek Craynor is almost eighty-nine years of age.

'He eats anything and everything', said his wife Rene, 'Sugar Puffs or jam butties for breakfast, sandwiches for lunch, and meat and two veg for the evening meal.'

Derek's fare is little different from that of anyone else in this study, except that they don't eat the Sugar Puffs. Lynn Ward and her mother who is 94 like a glass of Merlot. When pushed, most of the rest of my characters will also admit to liking a tipple with their evening meal. This is not much different from what they were serving the people in Pompeii: alcohol was nearly always served with their baked cheese and honey.

All of my characters like to eat out, all eat moderately and none of them are fussed with going on diets. Vic Trainer, our piranha fisherman, said that his metabolism was almost static.

'I just don't burn off the calories any more,' he said.

Joe Heathcote said 'It's the hardest exercise in the book, pushing yourself away from the table.'

The equivalent to that in Japan is hara hachi bu – eat moderately. In Okinawa people live ten years longer than most people on the planet. If you look at the people in our case studies, just swap the rice of the Japanese for our potatoes. They also pickle their vegetables and eat a lot of fish, including sushi. They too in Japan call it street food. They also like eel grilled over charcoal. They like their slices of beef, dried seaweed, chicken and pork, not quite as outlandish as tarantula or fried grasshopper but still street food or the food of the land.

Rich or poor, on the other side of the world or just down at St Osmund's in Bolton, Lancashire, it really makes little difference: just eat moderately, have a glass of wine for the stomach's sake and take some exercise.

HISTORY, KNOWLEDGE AND THE FUTURE

Malcolm Gladwell is an English-born Canadian journalist. He is also an excellent author of best selling books including 'The Tipping Point 'and 'Outliers', a book about success. One of his most cited quotations is from his book Blink, a story about making decisions. Gladwell says that we as human beings have a problem with telling stories: we are too quick to come up with explanations for things we don't really know too much about or an explanation that has no foundation. Diet is now a great topic for people to write books or articles about and build television shows around. In other words diet is hot. Book articles and TV shows all sell ideas and not all ideas have substantial foundations.

I started the charade at the age of fifteen. There were no diets then, no protein supplements, not even vitamin tablets. In those days I found it difficult to put on weight on my rather bony frame. I used to buy skimmed milk powder by the hundred weight, purchase Glaxo's Casilan and mix it with the whole milk to raise the fat levels. I remember reading about a brand of unsaturated vegetable oil, so I would add a few spoons of that to boost the fat content. By adjusting and selecting the right foods I could take my weight up and down.

The reason I learned to do this was to compete in lifting competitions. I perfected it so that I could lift in three different categories within weeks of each other. I weightlifted and entered bodybuilding competitions. This way for nearly twenty years I mastered weight control. It did nothing for my health but it was a great experience and sound knowledge to pass on. Now, half a century later, I have a different battle to fight, namely staying active in old age. Most of what I learned is useless for me now but I do understand the dynamics of it for the average punter out there. We don't need diets. We just need some common sense and a mind of our own.

Now it is a different story, Vic Trainer's metabolism is almost static and so is mine. Even in my forties it was difficult to strike that balance. My earlier days of lifting had given way to distance running and I had fancied having a go at running from John O'Groats to Land's End. There was a rather hazy world record of just over ten days, that meant running eighty miles a day, an unachievable goal as I would find out early in the run. Still I was running seventy miles a day and covered over five hundred miles in the eight days before losing my will, my heart and my bottle. At the age of forty-six I was to learn one of the most important lessons of my life.

CALORIES IN ENERGY OUT

It is estimated that we lose approximately one per cent efficiency per year after forty. Everyone is slightly different, so the slowing down process will vary with each individual. At forty-six I was probably ten per cent slower, ten per cent less efficient with my metabolism and ten per cent less able to sustain energy levels. It would be logical to assume that my body would need two to three thousand calories a day to cope with my seventy miles a day running. Not this time, in fact I actually put on eight pounds of body weight in the course of those eight days. Yes a pound a day. Eight, nine or even ten hours a day running and still I put on weight, a complete reversal from my early days of lifting weights. The reason was that to sustain my energy levels I need to keep my calories high, but I had problems eating regular food and still keeping on the move. This meant that my calorie intake was restricted to simple carbohydrates, mainly fruit cake. There was also a lot of pressure from the media, with BBC Television tracking me each and every day. People would also come out to run with me: such enthusiasm from supporters was both gratifying and touching but it did add pressure. There is only so much we can give without falling apart. It wasn't that, however, that sapped my strength and my resolve: it was sheer exhaustion and a very badly inflamed achilles tendon and, I suppose, the currant cake.

We learn not so much from our successes as from our failures and so it was from the John O'Groat's run. The run taught me that all the planning in the world will fail if we run out of steam, that pain and fatigue will make cowards of us all and that food is just a small part of the complexities of life. The secret to life's activities is not about diet or the kind of exercise, but our mental approach to diet and exercise. I had spent nearly a year specifically training for the run, plus thirty years of training and studying performance-related competition. Everything I had taken up, I competed in: swimming, soccer, weightlifting, bodybuilding and running. I have a desire and drive to excel even when I have no talent for the sport or pastime. I still have that desire and that drive and experience, and now after all these years there is a measure of understanding that didn't exist in my early years.

Food sustains us through life; we have a planet that provides. Rice in the eastern regions and potatoes, bread and wheat in the west. The oceans will provide all of us with fish. The people of the mountains will eat goat, pork or venison;

we have beef from the plains. Science, refrigeration, transportation and sophisticated storage ensures that no-one should starve and all of us survive. With reasonable healthy activity throughout and a mind that is not of someone else but our own, we will live off the land, shop at the supermarket, choose what we need and not necessarily what we want. We live on a self-sustaining planet with the intelligence to survive and prosper.

FOOD

Life expectancy across the world is not governed by the food of the country but by the conditions of the country. In the polar regions where people survive on fish, seal, and even polar bear, they will often eat their meat raw. They eat meagre amounts of fruit and vegetables, with the fish giving them copious amounts of omega 3. They have a life expectancy that is ten years less than the UK. That has little to do with their eating habits and more to do with the environment. They also lack good medical care and they have a higher rate of death at birth. The same can be said of tribes across the world. The Mexican running tribes have a wonderful regime of fitness and their eating habits are based around grain, with little meat and moderate amounts of fruit and veg. Their environment, however is harsh, unforgiving and like the Inuit, relentlessly difficult. Their environment and eating habits are like the eating habits that we have in the chapter on Billy Leach. They also have a lot of similarities to the people of Cambodia and Vietnam. Longevity is not so much about what we eat but more about where we live. In my town of Bolton, people will live longer by ten years by just not living in areas of deprivation. Food is not an issue here, but the amount and the choice is.

All of the people in the case studies in this book eat moderately: they are frugal without being conscious of being frugal. Their fare is different from that in Cambodia, but no more or less nourishing. They have found a balance of exercise and good eating habits and that is just one of the secrets to eternal youth regardless of where you live.

15 – SLOWING DOWN

We effectively start to slow down in our twenties. This very often levelled out if we exercise regularly. When reaching fifty, there is usually a marked change. It has been calculated that we lose 1% per year in all areas. Our strength, stamina, speed; the way we burn energy, our muscle tone and size. With regular exercise this can be slowed down. Concentration on specific areas can help this deterioration.

The natural law of ageing can never be halted but we can do an enormous amount to live and function well into our eighties and even nineties.

The secret to keeping it together is to keep moving and watch the intake of food. There is a lot to be gained by following the rules in the chapter 'Mind' in the section called 'Choices: We Are What We Think'.

The biggest challenge regardless of age is to keep it going – consistency – and all of the people in this book are great examples of this approach.

We should never lose sight of the four principles in the book:

Moderate Food

Constant Activity

Tribe

Feeding the Brain with Positive Affirmations

16 – MIND

Situated at the base of the skull and just above the spinal column is a cluster of cells called the Reticular Activating Systems (RAS). This part of the brain is no bigger than the circumference of a pencil yet it could have a huge part to play in how we shape our future.

Have you ever said 'It's been there in the back of my mind' or 'I remember the face but can't recall the name' or 'It's on the tip of my tongue'? Well that's the RAS in action. No part of the brain can work independently, so involving the RAS will also engage other groups and structures of the three pounds of grey matter, but it is the RAS that holds the key to training the brain.

This is not a great deal different to training ourselves to perform physical disciplines and comes down to simple repetition. Musical instruments, sport, military drills, education or just learning to drive a car, all of these things and many more are dependent on engaging our conscious mind to perform substantially. In other words, we learn to do things automatically. Training is about defining the specifics and continually refining the disciplines.

The RAS can act as a store to hold information to be triggered when needed. The soldier is expected to face death, the athlete to suffer pain, the musician to embrace harmony, the Formula One driver to remain cool at two hundred miles per hour or the student to think clearly when taking exams. All these rely on a trained and disciplined mind to come up with results when needed.

THE MIND SET

Growing older and staying younger is in simple terms the practice of staying younger. Research and scientific studies reveal that most people show their age too soon. Ageing is a process, a journey and the decline in age has little to do with how we feel but has a great deal to do with how we think. The process of ageing therefore is for the mind and this book shows just how important it is to being energised and active in those declining years.

Most people don't think about age until something happens to make them think about age. This can be triggered by an unexpected death at a relatively young age, or it may be an illness or an accident to ourselves, or a shock diagnosis that pulls us up short and prompts the thought 'Surely not me?'

How many times have we heard the sayings 'We are as young as we feel' or 'Age is in the mind'. It's paradoxical, according to Andy Rooney who said that the idea of living a long life appeals to everyone but the idea of getting old doesn't appeal to anyone.

The idea of writing this book came to me in my mid-seventies, but I felt that I wasn't old enough so I left it till I was eighty. Now, after researching and meeting so many ageing people and some wonderful and amazing characters, I wish I had started when I was younger which would have given me more time to enjoy the ageing process. The truth of the matter is that this journey didn't start when I was eighty.

LEUKAEMIA IN CHILDREN, GOING DAFT AT 40 AND HOW A SMALL BUNCH OF CELLS CHANGED MY LIFE

In fact, my journey started when I was fifteen years of age and serving my time as an apprentice bricklayer. I don't recall the name of the hospital, but I do remember the children's ward because everyone in that ward had leukaemia. The oldest child was about twelve and the matron said to me that none of the thirty or so patients would reach twenty years of age.

My boss that day was called Cliff Marsh. 'Go and get some water,' he said, giving me the bucket. So off I went. The only tap I could find was in the ward where all these children were and that turn of events would prompt me to do crazy things on my fortieth birthday, twenty-five years later.

That small group of cells called The Reticular Activating System had stored that memory for all of that time. So at the age of forty I decided I wanted to raise money for child leukaemia. I decided to do a series of endurance events that coincided with my fortieth birthday. It seemed fitting that whatever I was going to do related to my age, so it was logical to do a run of forty miles. I knew it was crazy to follow that with something else related to my age, so I decided to do a circuit of exercises with weights and set a target of forty thousand pounds in forty minutes. I still didn't think that was enough, so I came up with the idea of playing four people at squash, then finishing the day with four hundred sit ups.

I should also point out that, forty years ago, the age of forty was considered to be middle age, or even older. So to run forty miles, lift forty thousand pounds and play four people one after the other, plus do four hundred sit-ups was perhaps tempting fate too much. And perhaps it was. However, it did raise a considerable amount for child leukaemia. I had dragged a thought from the depths of my mind, a crazy exercise that started me on a journey that defied ageing and mastered a principle called mind over matter.

The memory of those kids when I was fifteen years of age was the catalyst to change my outlook on life. I had lifted weights and competed both as a lifter and a bodybuilder and now at the age of forty I had suddenly become an endurance athlete. Power and endurance are not the best of pals but somehow I transcended that gap and all because of that little thought in the back of my mind twenty-five years earlier.

GOING WHERE THE FISH FEED, GIVING YOURSELF A CRACK ON THE OTHER ELBOW AND WHY WE NEED MORE THAN ONE REASON TO ACHIEVE OUR GOALS

Bill Pearl is now eighty-six years of age. He is one of the greatest authorities on weight training in the world. Bill is a four times Mr Universe winner, a Mr America and holds among many other titles that of the World's Best-Built Man. He also collects cars, all kinds of cars. He has among his collection two 1920s Ford Model Ts, a Rolls Royce, a Lincoln Continental, and a vintage Ford Mustang. When Bill had used up all his space to store these cars he started to look at vintage bicycles. His enthusiasm doesn't stop there: he is the author of eight best-selling books and still owns a gym on his ranch in Oregon that is frequented by bodybuilders from all over the state. He is a Native American and one of the nicest men you could meet. He and his wife Judy live near the town of Talent, just off the Oregon Trail, the scene for so many westerns made in Hollywood.

In the year 1980, my business partner Bill Stevenson and I brought Bill Pearl to do a tour of England and to lecture on the benefits of exercise. The tour would also create an opportunity to promote his first book Keys to the Inner Universe. It was on one of the seminars that someone asked him a rather innocuous question.

The question was 'What do you do with a shoulder bursa?'

Bills answers to that was 'Give yourself a crack on the other elbow'.

Anyone who has trained over many years knows that training through injuries is a part of life, but the rather casual answer to a rather innocuous question goes much deeper than we think. Taking the mind out of the pain by inflicting pain elsewhere has a lot to do with success in other things. Finding a reason to keep going is about dividing and diverting the conscious and the subconscious. One way of doing this is to find more than one reason to do what you want to do. For me, becoming an endurance athlete at forty was not about doing feats of endurance but more about those children with leukaemia. When I have climbed mountains, swum in lakes, lifted weights or run to extreme lengths, it has not been about the physical effort but about raising money for kids fighting cancer, or seeing other people benefit, not just about satisfying my ego. Split, or even triple your motives to achieve your goals. So thinking young could only be one of the reasons for staying young.

There is a saying that if you want to fish then go where the fish feed. Learning from people like Bill Pearl was about going to the best source of information. The fact that we got to know each other personally and became lifelong friends was just a simple extension of our first meeting in 1969. When I started to research this book I needed to find people who knew more about ageing than I did. Meeting people like John Higson, Derek Craynor and all the people from the Fitness League was not just about information but more about learning about people and what makes them tick and, just as importantly, making friends and enjoying the process and the journey. I started out fishing for information and finished with an important development in my life which in turn gave me more insight into what helps people to really be active into old age.

It's not only about food, it's not about exercise: it's about tribe; it's about mind. Yes, we need to be conscious about food. Yes, we do need to be active. Yes, the type of food and activity play their part but the secret is in the company we keep and our attitude to life. Who knows how far we can go if all of us want to go to the same place.

OUT OF THE MOUTHS OF THE 70 YEAR OLD BABES

Mary McDaid, from County Wicklow in southern Ireland, said it:

'We don't just lead a class, we teach it. We also teach the brain: the left side of the brain and the right side of the brain. The left side of the brain means that they have to remember the moves that we have taught them. The right side of the brain copes with balance and posture, picking up the cues from the teacher and keeping pace with the music. It's important that they have to think of the past and to think of the now. The left side and the right side of the brain!'

Some scientists may argue with Mary, but not me. Mary and I were discussing this over breakfast. Well she was having a full English breakfast and I was sitting there, trying to keep up with this 67 year old teacher.

'Diet's important', she said, chewing on a piece of bacon, 'but we're not manic about it'

She went on to say how important friendship was. She recalled a time when one of her class had brought along a sick friend just to watch. They were friends, so why not bring someone who might benefit from watching the class. I don't suppose that Mary McDaid knows too much about the theory of psychology but I'm absolutely convinced that she is practising it.

One of the first things that Sam Allardyce did when he joined Bolton Wanderers Football Club was to employ Phil Brown as his assistant. Phil and I had talked many times about how important psychology was to sport. Even at that time in the late nineties, it was becoming obvious to me that soccer would embrace the philosophy. Psychology would have a part to play in the sport. Sam Allardyce is not a good manager: he is a great manager. Apart from his huge presence, his knowledge and his capacity for change, he also has great curiosity. Everything and anything that will improve performance is always worth looking at. It was no surprise to me that Sam would look into improving performance through psychology.

Sam's appointment of Mike Ford in 1999 started with a phone call from our son, Paul. 'There's a seminar at Preston North End,' he said, 'and the two guys who are delivering are Mike Ford and Mike Finnegan. Their company is called Advanced Training and they specialise in psychology in business and sport.' Both Phil Brown and I went to the breakfast seminar and Phil later took his report back to manager Colin Todd. Colin left the club soon after this but had agreed to bring Advanced Training in on a trial basis, little knowing that his departure was imminent. It did not take long for Sam Allardyce to appoint Mike Ford to be Bolton's in house sports psychologist. It also heralded a decade of quite magical football.

Just how important psychology is to football was demonstrated when Sam Allardyce left for pastures new. Mike Ford was put on garden leave until the appointment of the new manager and was eventually released. Within days, Mike Ford was employed by Chelsea FC under the management of José Mourinho. I think that psychology is ever present in us in that we follow a path in life that leads us to search for a more stable and safe existence. When Sam Allardyce managed Bolton Wanderers, he led a Tribe of people who made up his following. They were searching for stability and a safer journey as were the people who eventually voted him out. The soccer fan wants leadership and a leader who provides stability and safety for the future. People follow people who provide a path to a future.

GREAT THINGS HAPPEN WHEN PHYSIOLOGY AND PSYCHOLOGY MEET

It is now over a hundred years since William James stated that the greatest discovery of his generation was that human beings could alter their lives by altering their attitudes of mind.

It has taken over a century to name the concept and we now call it neuroplasticity. Another great mind of the past, Albert Einstein, said

'It is all out there: there is nothing new, we just have to find ways to find it" and many of the people in this book have found it.

Neuroplasticity means that we can remould the brain to change our lives. Edward Taub, Norman Doidge, Michael Merzenich and countless other highly-respected doctors and scientists are forging the way forward in not just improving our minds, but scientifically curing disablement from strokes, Alzheimer's Disease and even forms of blindness.

Edward Taub is a Behavioural Neuroscientist at the University of Alabama. He is best known for his major break-throughs in neuroplasticity and discovering and developing constraint-induced movement therapy, a collection of techniques that help stroke victims recover the use of their paralysed limbs.

Constraint-induced movement therapy means that the affected limb is made to work by performing special exercises. In the case of an affected arm, only that arm would be made to function. The unaffected arm would be left immobile, not unlike Bill Pearl's giving yourself a crack on the other elbow. Pearl and Taub are about the same age: both have been at the top of their professions. Taub's academic career is unsurpassed and so is Pearl's: one is driven by scientific study, the other by doing.

Taub is recognised for his therapy which will undoubtedly enhance the recovery of stroke victims, Alzheimer's cases and brain-damaged patients. His techniques of concentrating on the affected arm, forces the brain to find a way to make the arm or limb work. As in all training, we have to be constant. Consistency and repetitive work gives the brain little option and by not having options the brain finds new ways to work the limb. Science calls this developing new neural pathways and thus neuroplasticity evolved.

Dr. Wendy Suzuki, a neuroscientist at New York University, is pioneering brain connection and development by asking class participants to use their minds when doing aerobic exercise. Such self-affirmation involves consistently repeating positive thoughts, goals and visualising images in the mind. What Dr. Suzuki is saying is what Mary McDaid was saying to me over eggs and bacon. Is this why the Fitness League has such old participants? Mary, like thousands of her colleagues, keeps active because she has to think, act, deliver complicated moves, and at the same time, teach and observe others. Here we have two entirely different approaches by two people. One is a neuroscientist and the other a woman running an exercise class for thirty people in a church hall in County Wicklow. In reality they are both saying the same thing.

Norman Doidge is a psychiatrist, a psychoanalyst, and a

New York Times bestselling author. His book The Brain that Changes Itself sold over a million copies and was chosen by the Dana Foundation's journal Cerebrum as the best general book in English ever written on the brain.

Doidge, like Taub, Suzuki and many others is pioneering a new era in curing disablement through the power of the mind. Sylvia Faucitt, Derek Craynor, Billy Leach and many more have actually been practising these basic self-affirmations throughout their six, seven or eight decades of living. When Sylvia Faucitt fell and broke her neck she had her own self-affirmations already in place.

'I don't look for excuses to stop: I look for reasons to continue.' This is a state of mind brought about by the constant use of exercise and by a way of life. Derek Craynor, like many others, refuses to take medication except in extreme cases. His exercise programmes over the last seventy-odd years have built a fortress of impregnability. There are hundreds of women in the Fitness League who ritualistically practise well-rehearsed and choreographed exercise that creates and stimulates the body and the brain. All the people in this book are merging the physiology and psychology: they are by design practising the principles of mind and body and by accident reinforcing the principles of neuroplasticity.

The psychology of sport is no different from the psychology of politics or government or the psychology of exercise. Each and every one of us is searching for a safer path to follow and a journey through life. The England team members in soccer list their faith in the last leader and now search for victory under the new leader. The voters in the Brexit referendum had lost faith in the leaders of Europe. We will all continue to follow the pioneers in neuroplasticity: Edwards Taub, Wendy Suzuki, Norman Doidge, Mary McDaid and the other people in this book because they provide us with a promise of a better future, a more stable and secure path to follow in living the life we live.

CHOICES: WE ARE WHAT WE THINK

There are few more important things in life than our health. Some may argue that love precedes all: the love for another, the love for our family, or the love of a cause worth fighting for. Victor Frankl in his book Man's Search for Meaning says that there is no greater cause than the love of mankind and, if that is so, then it is a cause worth dying for.

In the early nineteen eighties the business guru Tom Peters said in his book 'In Search of Excellence' that there is no reality, only perception. If we think it is there in our minds, it is. Both Frankl and Peters were singing off the same sheet: our lives are governed by how we see things in life and what we see can only be interpreted by our thoughts. Everything we see, touch, smell, hear or presume is a simple result of what we think. That cream bun, packet of crisps, vitamin supplement or exercise class is what we see or perceive and our choice or choices are decided by our mind.

At the age of nineteen, I was one of many millions of males who were conscripted in the armed forces. I had little thought on the matter; it was a government decision and therefore law. So off I went to be a soldier. The soldier is not allowed to think too much. So much of what the soldier does he just does, but even in our armed forces we are allowed choices provided it is for the betterment of all. One of the betterment choices was to volunteer for a specialist group. I thought it a good idea at the time, so put my name forward for the parachute regiment. The Special Forces pay better money and that half of my mind pressed the cash register while the other part of my mind played possum.

It is said that there are only two sure things in life: death and taxes. Everything else is subject to how we look at life. My near two years in the Paras taught me a lot of things, not the least being that our minds are more easily shaped at a younger age. At nineteen, death is less of a reality, and that is why the armed forces throughout the world are predominantly made up of the young. There is a lot of wisdom in the saying that old soldiers never die, they just fade away. One lesson that has stayed with me for over sixty years was learned by my Para training, and that is by constant drills we become robots. In other words, we do things without thought. Drills, practised movement and constant repetition washes the brain: we act automatically and leap out of a plane into nothingness because of the constant repetitive drills that programme the perfect exit. Athletes know this, soccer managers should know this, the ballet teacher and all who become leaders of others coax, cajole, bully and exercise their subtle persuasions to get what they want.

In the early nineteen fifties the publishing company Penguin released a rather insignificant book called The Hidden Persuaders by Vance Packard. Packard's specialty was writing about human behaviour and in The Hidden Persuaders, he wrote about how the public in America and Britain were being brainwashed into buying goods and commodities through marketing techniques that came under the heading of subliminal persuasion.

All this was at a time when the large supermarkets were being built across the States. Motivational behaviour was a top subject in universities and colleges and large funds were available to develop and discover new ways to sell consumer goods. This was also a time when television was invading the home and Hollywood films were at their peak. Both the small and large screen were ideal vehicles for selling through the subconscious mind.

Part of Packard's book explains how subliminal marketing works on our vulnerable minds. There are eight hidden persuaders all of which involve our need for security. Exercise, food and tribe are all agents for boosting our thoughts to protect. Our hierarchy of needs changes with the times. In the fifties everyone was vulnerable as we were still recovering from two world wars. Food, clothing and fuel were just a few of the things that we needed. One of the big sellers at the time was the freezer, a commodity that ensured our supply of food. Air conditioning was another target. Air conditioning meant closed windows, doors and particularly at night, keeping everything at night neat: a safer home. There were other goods that the psychologists would target in influencing and persuading people's minds and controlling what we think.

The recovery from World War II saw a whole new way of doing things. It would be the start of the mass markets. The supermarkets and television would lead the charge with cars and travel to follow. Automation and mass-produced goods would open the door to world trade and with that a huge change in how we perceived security. The coal industry would all but disappear; manufacturing would go to all regions of the planet; shipbuilding in both Britain and America would be greatly reduced; changes in the cotton and wool industries would all add to our anxieties and unemployment would change our behavioural patterns for ever.

Every time we have change in our lives we have differences of thought. All of us believe that we make decisions that benefit us individually but in truth we are all influenced by others. Even the great leaders are surrounded by experts who in turn act and advise on the advice of others. We are what we think but the choices we make are anything but our own.

The saving grace in all of this is that we do still have choices. We can choose our mode of activity and what food we eat and we can choose the company of others and feel safe and comfortable in our choice of tribe. We should all be careful, however, that what we think are our thoughts are indeed the thoughts of our mind and not being influenced by the thoughts of others. How will we ever know?

The psychology of living longer and still remaining active will always be a challenge, not for the body but for the mind. We are what we think because everything we do starts with our thoughts and therefore with what we choose.

17 – BRAIN

In 1988 The Institute of Human Knowledge published a book called The Healing Brain by Robert Ornstein and David Sobel. Ornstein, a professor of Human Biology and Sobel, a director of preventative medicine, wrote between them more than fourteen books about the same subject. The Healing Brain discounted most of what we call medicine and credited thought and good habits as being the way forward.

Fast forward two and a half decades and we have another book by Dr Norman Doidge, a highly acclaimed book on the same subject called The Brain that Changes Itself, about a revolutionary subject called neuroplasticity. Both of these two books, twenty-five years apart, argue the same points, the difference between the two being that Doidge's book is now backed by conclusive proof that we can indeed change ourselves both physically and mentally by thought.

Neuroplasticity is the brain's ability to reorganise itself by forming new neural connections throughout life. It allows the neurons in the brain to compensate for injury and disease and to adjust activity in response to new situations or to changes in environment.

Ornstein and Sobel got it right in 1988 but it took the last twenty-five years to prove that we have it in us to heal, change our thoughts, actions, habits, character and even our destiny.

This book started out with a totally different objective to how it finished. My whole adult working life has been devoted to developing the physical part of our existence and now among other things I am writing about the brain.

There is hardly any sport that I have not been involved in: soccer, rugby, athletics, swimming, basketball, bodybuilding, weight-training and weight-lifting, and even training chess players to improve their concentration. Now by default I am writing about the trillions of cells, neurons, synapses, neural pathways and what science now calls neuroplasticity.

The mind has always been instrumental in training the body. Competing in sport, even in nurturing people just to become fitter, to slim or look good on the beach or for that special occasion. But now it's different. Things have changed. It is no longer enough to be involved with the psychology, the motivational implications of winning, losing or achieving goals. It is no longer enough to know what happens. We now want to know why and how and just what is going on in the functional organ called the brain.

For this I once more turned to the world's leading experts on the subject, the latest phase in a hundred years of study. I turned to Michael Merzenich and his book Soft Wired, written in the language of the layman. That and a stack of similar literature tells us what's going on in that wonderful and marvellous part of our being called the brain. A moveable feast of manipulative matter.

As strange as it may seem, developing the brain is not unlike developing our physical prowess. Our bodies need to be challenged and to keep improving performance we need to keep raising the bar. The muscles of our bodies become accustomed to a certain level of activity and so it is with the brain. The brain, like the body, will deteriorate over time and, unless we keep it fresh, it deteriorates quicker. Keeping the brain in shape is dependent on regular mental exercise combined with regular exercise for the body.

The mind is the software, the brain the hardware. The mind is the goal-setter, the brain is the goal-getter. The three and a half pounds of grey matter is the executor of the strategists: one action, the other thought. All of it is protected by a thin layer of bone known as the skull. The average mature brain is approximately six inches long and contains one hundred billion cells. There is more power than in all the world's armies put together, all the computers on the planet, and all the untapped wisdom of all governments across all lands. The divisions of the brain form the nervous system's cerebrum, hippocampus, hypothalamus, cerebral and frontal lobes and with all its divisions it is not unlike the high command of the mind.

So how does that communication work? How do we get the message across? How will the brain respond to what we 'the mind' want it to do? In answer to that we need to go no further than the example of the armed forces or all the computers across the world. In simple terms you send the message out via the communication channels and make your intentions clear. The armed forces will send the message out through their networks first through the Intelligence Department then through the signal divisions and through the network of higher and lower commands. If you want to access the hardware of your computer then you develop the software and feed it into the system. The system then is dependant on the connectors: your database, social media, and how many you can reach across all your repertoire of people.

In all cases, armies, companies or social networking, it is the clarity of the message that counts. In our case, it is to challenge the brain to reshape itself and extend the efficiency of our mental capacity. A sound mind in a sound body. The brain's method of communicating this message starts with the nervous system: the frontal lobe, parietal, temporal and occipital lobes. Messages and pathways are formed. There are literally hundreds of millions of cells and neurons hungry to be challenged, desperate to be engaged and wonderfully receptive to your efforts.

Scientists across the world are all too aware that our brains shrink with age. There is little doubt in Merzenich's book Short Wired that in order to help prolong our mental agility we need to continually challenge the brain. New skills, mental concentration, physical exercise, learn something new each day, be it academic or a new physical skill, everything helps replace those dead cells with new ones.

The reality of this hit home watching Ann Hunt lead the class at St Osmund's. The level of concentration in each of those seventy, eighty and even ninety year olds was testament to Mary McDaid's quote: 'We train the left and right side of the brain'. and to Ewan Kelly's observation about being there, concentrating and not just going through the motions. All this entails a sense of purpose, a place to be, a bowling green, an exercise class, an alert mind when hiking, walking or swimming. Vic Trainor's attitude and Derek Craynor's consistency and his desire to just keep going come to mind as do thoughts of an active mind in an active body and a brain that accepts the fact that to rest is to rust. An attitude of mind comes from within, as our friend Billy Leach said to me over forty years ago.

UNVEILING THE BRAIN: THE LAYMAN'S TERMS

Nothing happens without the brain's say so and there is no one part of the brain that works independently without millions or even trillions of neurons and brain cells contributing to the end result, whatever that may be.

The large cluster of neurons of the cortex sits above the thalamus, the centre of the brain. Information is relayed to various parts via the ganglia, a group of structures that are involved in voluntary movement. The limbic system is responsible in part with our emotions, something that Steve Peters called the chimp factor in his book Mind Management. This is often called the reptilian brain and includes the hippocampus, hypothalamus and amygdala. All of these influence memory. The mid-brain is a small area at the top of the brain and it is this small cluster of cells that deals with eye movement and is involved with the release of dopamine, a substance that lifts our emotions, give us the feel-good factor and is essentially nature's way of patting us on the back and saying well done. The adrenalin rush is triggered by all the things that keep up alive: food, water, sex, overcoming setbacks and importantly, challenge. If we are to replace the dying cells in our brain then we must cultivate the physicalities that prolong our existence: exercise, activity and being involved with others in the tribe. It really is quite simple and is illustrated in every chapter of this book and nowhere more obviously than in the chapter called People.

THE FITTEST OR THE STRONGEST?

This year I will celebrate, if that's the word, my eighty-second birthday. I have mentioned the feats of strength and endurance that I have achieved over the years. A 2:31 marathon at age 45, the charity events on my 40th and 50th birthdays. I have never been gifted with too much talent, something to do with lung function and fast twitch fibres in the muscles. Playing to my strengths was the answer or so I thought all those years ago and on reflection I was probably right. This year will be no exception: even now in my eighth decade it will be yet another challenge. Three open water swims, 5K in Lake Windermere will kick it off in June. The full length of Coniston is five miles and that will be done in July. Six weeks after Windermere. Then it will be time for the big one: the full length of Windermere, ten plus miles point to point. At eighty-two, a battle not with the water but with the mind.

There is always the other voice that wants out; one voice saying this needs to be done, three, four, five or six miles in the pool; the level of concentration, a single- minded approach and a conscience that says put it off till Tuesday, Wednesday or Thursday. The battle rages and has done all of my life. First it was weight-lifting, never quite making the top but very credible poundages, not for want of commitment, not for want of desire, just short of a few of those genes. Running came easier until I came face to face with the gifted. Now the strength has faded, the legs have gone the way of all flesh and it's the water that tempts the ghosts of the ambitious past. The saving grace is that I loved it, wallowed in it, embraced the not quite good enough, not the failure, but the striving, the straining, the battles and wars and all the sheer pumping of the adrenalin and dopamine. The sheer exhilaration of a 275 pound clean and jerk, a personal best in a 10 mile, 10K or the ultimate twenty-six miles, three hundred and sixty- five yards: endorphins, serotonin and the psychological triumph of mastering self. It is not the fastest or the strongest, but the ones that adapt said Darwin and everyone in this book is an example of the great philosopher's wisdom.

It is now forty years since Billy Leach first said that our health comes from within. Just how that can be explained is no clearer now than it was then. Perhaps Billy was talking about our minds, a belief or obscure mantra from the lips of a sage, monk or other holy man from the mountains of Tibet but not from the coal miner in Lancashire. Regardless of its origin, we now know that this is no mere philosophy but a simple function of the bunch of cells in the hippocampus, controlled not by some mystical invisible entity but by how hard you work at the grey matter we call the brain.

BRAIN TRAINING

When did it start? Was it at the end of the Industrial Revolution or was it a result of the age of television? Was it all about the inception of technology and the digital age? Whatever the reason, dementia is becoming the modern day plague. The dying cells that effect memory, movement and reasoning are a major issue for now and for the foreseeable future.

Coordination, thinking the way through problems, physically changing the way we work, calculation without a calculator, plotting our journeys and not relying on the sat nav are ways of using the brain. In the past we listened to the radio, engaging our imagination. We shopped at the butcher's, the baker's, the grocer's and greengrocer's. We read newspapers, walked to the telephone kiosk, observed and used time to calculate the things we could see. We walked to the cinema, the market shops, the football matches, the playing fields, the swimming pool and the park. We walked to church, the youth club, the gym, to our friends' and neighbours' homes and to the pub. We played cards, dominoes, darts and engaged in conversation.

We had an unbelievable exchange of dialogue. There was little or no time to fill: our day was already full of opportunities to stop, talk with people along the way, on the bus, on the train, in the street or at work. We engaged our lives with so many things that our brains were continually on the go. As indeed were our bodies. Most if not all of this is now in the past. Asda, Tesco, Morrisons, Sainsburys and other supermarkets have replaced sparsely and strategically placed corner shops and the three-day open markets. The walk or journey by tram or bus is now replaced by conveniently-placed car parks with days spent shopping for oven-ready meals for two.

In go the plates, knives and forks, cups, saucers and pudding dishes, frying pans, or anything we can place in the automatic dish washer. No wringers or scrubbing boards. The endless washing line replaced in part by the high-tech spin dryer and non-iron materials manufactured for our convenience and labour-saving life, reducing the brain's desperate need to be challenged.

In 2017 we celebrate the early steps of the artificial brain cell implant for prosthetic limb movement by thought alone. A marvellous and astonishing revolution of how inventive we can be. It has always been on the cards. My childhood hero Wilson of the Wizard had unexplainable powers of the mind and mighty men from the Himalayas thawing themselves out of a block of ice slowing their heart rate to zero and going in and out of self-induced comas. Like the animals of the wild in hibernation, nature does have a way.

'There is nothing new' said Albert Einstein, 'It's all there; we just need to find it.'

For that we need the brain, curiosity, will power and desire. Difficult when the world we live in is driven by convenience.

PUTTING THE BRAIN TO WORK

There are thousands of neuroscientists across the world who are currently working on the brain's way of healing itself. Like all things in life, we have to work at getting the brain to do what we want it to do and the best way to do that is to work at it daily. For a good example of this just look at my case studies in the chapter on People. Len Russell who is coming up to ninety swims and talks his way though forty lengths a day. Ewan Kelly lifts heavy weights and hikes the local country-side keeping his brain functioning because he thinks when doing his exercise. Concentration is a major key, just ask

Mary McDaid or Sylvia Faucitt, or any of the women from the Fitness League.

"It's not rocket science" is a cliché but it's true in this case.

Professor Michael Merzenich will tell you to think about what you are doing, learn new skills, enter an age of discovery, change something having learned it, replace your bad habits with good ones and challenge yourself in dozens of small ways. Read the chapters on Zone, Place, and Ritual. If you're a walker shorten or lengthen your step and give your brain something to think about. Look for something new around the countryside or in familiar streets around you. Small challenges overcome big fears. Find some purpose, as did Tony Ford, Hamish McPherson and our friend Len Russell. His challenges like the guys in The Full Monty gave him a reason to live. Join a gym, try everything and remember the brain is just as important as the body. Like our heart, we need to use it, nurture it, and treat it with the respect it deserves.

I have now been prescribing exercise for nearly half a century. For forty of those years I did it for a living. The real beauty of what I did was that there was always something new around the corner. We had our competing athletes in abundance from bobsleigh to boxers but the real value was in the mothers of children, the recovering people who had had surgery or major illness and the ordinary people who had no knowledge of physical exercise. For over twenty years we trained the trainers, installing fundamental skills on correct delivery, breathing techniques and importantly how to gain the confidence and trust of the client. Good coaches develop instincts for what is right, they engage the mind of the client and deliver a belief. They praise and reprimand, cajole and even bully and know when to press the right button. They know when to push and when not, and like Sylvia Faucitt not to make excuses but to find the right reasons to go on.

That is what the brain is looking for. It is looking for you to be coached and use your lifetime instincts to keep going. The brain needs to be guided: think positive, take a leaf from Derek Craynor, Billy Leach, Vic Trainer, and Sally Floyd and train the brain like you would or should train the body. Set goals, not big ones, but lots of small ones. Len Russell swims five days, one of his goals is to never miss, another goal is to do forty lengths. Tony Ford's daily bowling sessions and two holidays a year playing bowls in Cyprus are short term and long term goals. Hamish McPherson now in his ninety-first year hates missing his three workouts a week at the gym. Hamish's eyes won't allow him to drive so he catches the bus. These people set themselves goals and challenges, they know the value of ritual, they don't want to miss a session: the challenges and goals send messages to the brain and it responds.

Brain training is not a science, it is an everyday occurrence and it is in the chapters of this book that you can find the secrets to keeping the brain active. Every chapter was penned from the interviews, secrets that people didn't even know they had hidden away in the lockers of their minds. The real secret was that they engaged their minds to talk to their brains.

18 – PEOPLE

'It's elementary, Dear Watson,' said Holmes. 'Elementary!'

The deductive powers of Sherlock Holmes were all down to the creativity of Arthur Conan Doyle who could, through his imagination and writing skill, conjure up any solution he wished.

I knew from the start that the answer to my conundrum would not come from my mind or from my ability to write a satisfying ending. The answers would come from the people of this book. Sir Arthur Conan Doyle penned some great stories that have excited us for generation. Holmes is still in the cinema and on television.

This story, however, is far different from a one-off crime or then again, maybe not; for obesity, dementia, Alzheimer's, Parkinson's and the other related diseases are just as dastardly as the characters in the fictitious tales of Mr Conan Doyle. This time the stories are real, the people are real and certainly the modern plague is real.

The mystery started, as I recall, on the second visit to St Osmund's church hall. This was to set up some interviews. It didn't take long to realise that I too had a mystery.

'You have something here,' I said to Ann Hunt, 'and I can't figure it out. It's like everyone is thinking the same, eating the same, talking the same.'

I remember using the word telepathy. Don't be daft, I thought, then immediately questioned it. Frustrated, I turned back to Ann and told her I would find the answer, and with that she looked at me puzzled then turned and went back to teaching her class. It was then that Lynn Ward came across and thrust into my hand a sheaf of notes, sheets of paper with information about her mother, Wynne, a member of the Fitness League since 1945.

Lynn said she had joined for the history and that left me even more baffled than before. Ten months later, my answers came and had nothing to do with deductive powers. The clues were already there and slowly, ever so slowly, they would emerge, sock me in the jaw, tell me to stop being stupid and listen to what all these people were saying.

What, I wondered, had history to do with the left or right side of the brain? What had a class of ageing women to do with a dance class in New York City thirty-eight years ago and with the choreographed lecture of Ann Hunt in a church hall at St Osmund's just one and a half miles away from my front door in Bolton? What had all the lines from all these people got to do with dementia? What wisdom would emerge from the mouths of these people: Ewan Kelly, Tony Ford, Mary McDaid in County Wicklow, Sylvia Faucitt, Alan Farnworth and all the others?

This was when I decided not to tell you anything. I would put you in my shoes and give you the chance to be lifted, moved and motivated by these ordinary people with some extraordinary gifts for living longer, being active and teaching us secrets to eternal youth. Listen to what they have to say, hear the wisdom of their mantras and their beliefs. Piece it together as I did, enjoy their humour, their individuality and their simplicity, and be prepared to challenge as I did because it is these people who shaped, directed and showed me how to connect the dots, form the chapters and see the beginning of the end.

Ewan Kelly

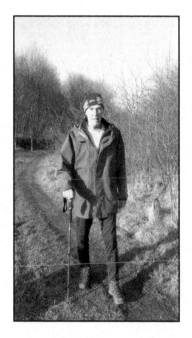

❝ *Two things are important; one is consistency and being in the present. It's no good just going through the motion, the mind needs to be on what you are doing.* **❞**

John Higson, 94

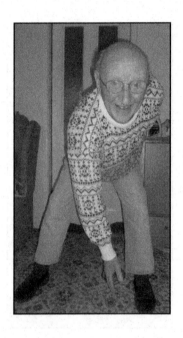

❝ *'I made my mind up when I was 24 that I would live to be a hundred. Now at 94 I still do my exercises and walk daily. Here's me touching my toes!'* **❞**

Vic Trainer, 77

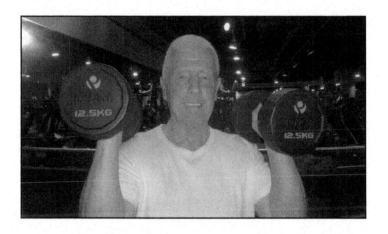

" *I am going up the Amazon fishing for piranha for my holidays.* "

Heidi Boyle, 76

Two days after the interview, Heidi told me that she had swum 21 miles in the health club pool.

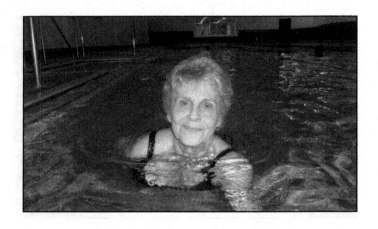

" *Oh, I forgot to tell you, I swam the channel.* "

Derek Craynor, 89

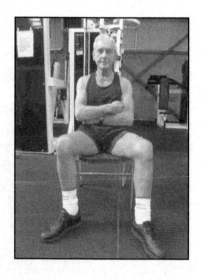

" *My Grandma used to tell me that when you rest you rust.* **"**

Hamish McPherson,
now over 90

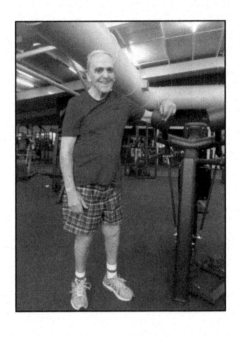

❝ *I used to like competing so I still work out with weights to fill the gap* **❞**

Len Russell, 87

Len says he keeps going because he
doesn't know how to give up.

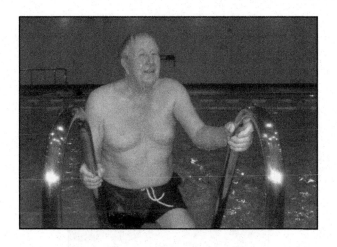

" *I have had four bypass surgeries, two replacement
knees, one stent and prostate surgery and I am still here.*

"

Sylvia Faucitt

Here she is 10 years after falling down
the stairs and breaking her neck.

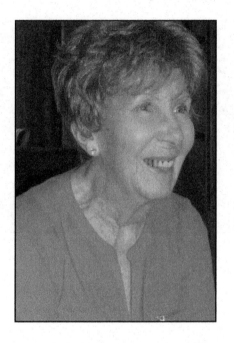

" *Some people look for excuses to stop; I look for reasons to keep going. I do Women's League, zumba, walk the dogs an a little exercise at home.* **"**

Joe Heathcote

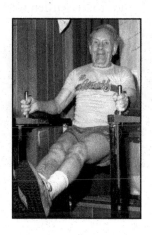

 The hardest exercise you will ever do is to push yourself away from the table before you are full.

Alan Farnworth, 90

Alan is a flat green bowler, who still plays
four times a week. He loves walking, and
still tends to his garden to this day.

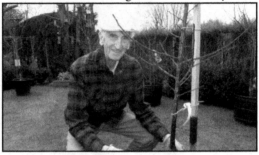

" *I lost my wife two years ago. I am restricted to certain
food because of a throat operation, so cooking came hard to
me. I play flat green bowls three times a week.* **"**

Mary McDaid

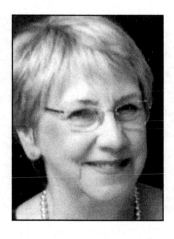

" We don't just lead the class, we teach them to remember the moves. So we are working the left side of the brain. Now when doing the class they have to follow me and pay attention to their posture, follow me and move to the music. So they are working the right side of the brain. "

Olga Brown, 80

Olga swims, does body conditioning, palates and water aerobics.

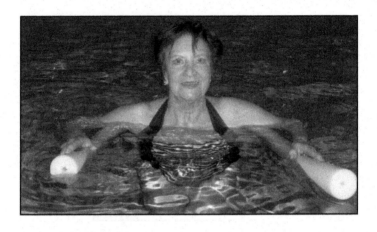

" *I do water aerobics, yoga and other classes. Life's about love, family and friends. We like music classical and jazz and the company of others.* "

Tony Ford, 85

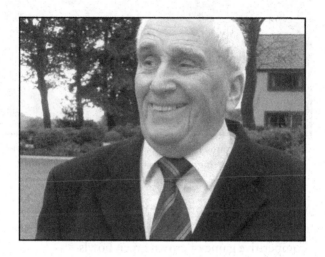

"" *I thought it was all over when my wife died; then someone introduced me to crown green bowls. I didn't like it at first but then I got hooked. That's seven years ago and I play nearly every day. I think I now know about two hundred people by their first name.* ""

Tony Ford's TRIBE at his local Crown Green Bowling Club:

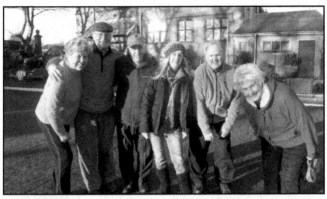

Left to right: Brenda Heathcote, Colin Makinson, Tony Ford, Margaret Turtington, Stuart Bailey, Joyce Makinson

Margaret Turtington took up bowls after a very active sporting background. She loves the friendship and the relaxed but competitive game of crown green bowls.

"My tribe is world wide: Holland, South Africa, New Zealand and Canada. The Fitness League saves peoples lives and is an antidote to loneliness."
– Lorna Kemp hails from Dublin. She values networking, friendship, laughter and yes, exercise.

"We change the choreography quite regularly it keeps them on their toes. The left and right side of the brain."
– Ann Hunt. Leader of the Bolton St Osmunds Fitness League

"When I exercise with The Fitness League I am always in a good place. The moves help our memory."
– Betty Brown, 73, after two knee replacements and breast cancer.

"We like the history because The Fitness League is proven, tested and reliable. Mother joined in 1945, she is now 94 and I am still doing it."
– Lynn Ward.

"I have taught ballet and aerobics now I teach Women's League and they can do this forever."
– Sally Floyd, who at 68 still teaches three classes per week in Edinburgh.

Margaret Brown, 70: never misses her exercise. She loves the companionship of The Fitness League, walks her dog, tap dances and loves the ritual.

96 year old Wynne Barber is Lynne Ward's mother and was in The Women's Army Core during the war. The Women's League of Health and Beauty was her return to sanity. She has now been a member for over 60 years and is only now showing signs of dementia.

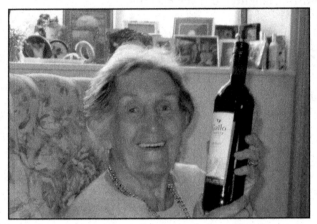

Wynne Barber 96, enjoying a glass of Merlot
with her tea-time fish and chips.

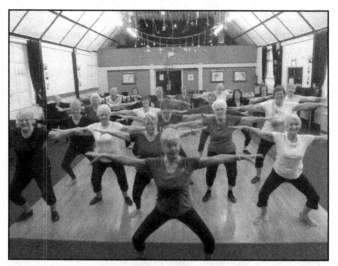

Here we have smiles, congeniality, friendship and we have TRIBE, purpose and perhaps we have all of the other chapters too.

Ann Hunt leading the class at St Osmond's Fitness League February 2017.

A combined total of 2192 years in her full class of 29 members.

(pictured with 21 members with a combined age of 1587)

This was when I saw the resemblance to the 70's Fame nearly 40 years ago. The women could easily be the age of the dancers from that television programme. This is what inspired the book.

When I asked Mary Clare how much exercise she did she said: *'Not enough'.*

Mary is now 88 years old, like her friend Sheila Wells, 86, exemplifies the ritual of The Fitness League.

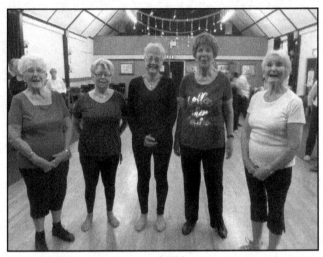

Left to right: **Mary Clare, Marian Berry, Lynn Ward, Sylvia Faucitt, Sheila Wells. Members of the St Osmund's Fitness League in Bolton**

"It wasn't teaching the classes, I still love to teach, it was just the sixty mile round trip and a half hour class was getting too much."

– Brenda Tone. What struck me was Brenda's attitude; she may have relinquished her teaching job but still at 75 continues to do her classes.

99% never mentioned the Mediterranean Diet, the Five a Day, nor did they take any form of supplements.

In the Fitness League: 93% said that friendship was the most important thing: TRIBE.

Only 3% of the people I met carried bottled water.

Bert Loveday was a Mr Britain at the age of 24. He was still bench pressing 200 lb at the age of 80, and played squash until his late 70s.

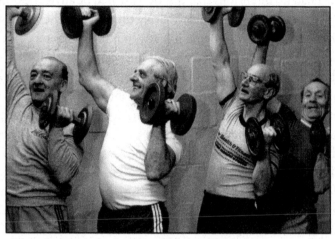

Left to right: Bert Loveday, Joe Wilson, Syd Baker and Joe Heathcote

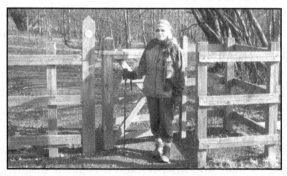

"Good health is the top and bottom of it. I hike, cycle, do Tai Chi, line dances and swim. I don't do the long walks any more; I just do up to 8 miles."
– Eileen Mary Bailey, 83.

All physically and mentally active. I just kept bumping into 90 year olds who still took part in regular exercise. Some said they didn't have alcohol but they had wine.

I had no intentions that this book would be anything other than about people who live actively till the end. There was no thought of obesity or dementia. My four main chapters would be: Activity, Psychology, Community and Diet. All four of these basic structures would still be in place but would all take on a different meaning. I didn't really interview people: it was more about sharing information. They changed the storyline, justified the chapters, and made sense of the narrative. Where the chapter on Stickiness came from was Len Russell's story about his four bypasses and his two knee replacements. He doesn't keep going because he needs to but because he wants to. And Dad's *'Don't do want you like, but like what you do'* inspired the chapters on Place and Choice.

'Be led by your gut' said Steve Jobs in our first chapter and it was these people that led my gut. It was these that set me my challenge and my choice of chapters. Each and every one and inspiration to me and I hope to you.

Most of them will keep popping up in the next few chapters, justifying the titles. You have here in this chapter just a few of the many hundreds of people out there who have similar stories and similar lives. All I would have to do was cast my net wider to find them. I have no doubt that I would get more of the same ordinary people, and their extraordinary knowledge. With the help of these people I believe that we have the power to overcome anything but we have to explore and look. We have to share and discover and it is in the discovery that enables us to change; and so it was with this book.

The change started with the remark from Lynn Ward, puzzling and innocuous. It was later at Lilleshall when Mary mentioned the right side of the brain and the left side that the penny dropped and then another one when Sally Floyd said *'They can do this forever.'* It would not be the final penny but it would be a significant one when Ann was leading the class to the tune of Sam Smith and I was on cloud nine travelling back in time and distance to New York in the late seventies.

'History,' said Lynn.
'Forever,' said Sally.
'If you rest you rust,' said Derek, and
'It comes from within' said Billy forty or fifty years ago.

Nine months into the study, sixty five years of searching and then that blinding flash of the obvious.

PEOPLE POWER

It would be eight months into the research and a hundred interviews and conversations before I realised that all the seventy, eighty and even the ninety year olds had no signs of dementia. Lynn Ward had told me that her mum, who is now 96, was showing signs. She doesn't do classes now but she still enjoys the family life, and her glass or two of Merlot. It was at this point that I became conscious that the book was going in a different direction. This is not, I thought, a book on keeping fit into old age, but a book about mental and physical agility into old age. So don't listen to me, listen to them because they will tell you that they have no secrets. It is quite elementary really. They just take it in their stride, keep it simple, don't eat too much and keep a good mental attitude. But of course that is what the chapters are about. Well they did tell me.

19 – STICKINESS

STICKINESS

Ask yourself what it is that you want. Do a little inventory of what it is that helps to keep your life on track. There is no simple answer nor should it be complicated. There is always a middle road but it does help to know what you want and to set yourself some little goals.

I was once talking to a stranger on the train going down to London. We found out that we had something in common. We were both into exercise. He swan and I ran. It was inevitable that we got onto injuries, probably the most common ground among athletes. Neither of us had had major injuries so in reality we were both talking about niggles and niggling injuries. Then he said something that has stuck with me for thirty years.

'I can't be doing with these niggles, I just tell them to go away and they do.'

Most people stop exercising because of little things, not because of major injuries. That statement from my friend on the train comes back to me more so now than any in other period in the past three decades. Perhaps age has taught me that the mind is far more powerful than I ever thought. I don't write goals down any more or keep a log but I am conscious of going where I want to go. I am even more aware now that I need a challenge and that these days, after nearly seven decades of working out, I need daily challenges and bigger challenges for the year. Each day I swim: my goal is five mornings per week. Like Ed Whitlow, I can find it a bit of a drag but I go not out of determination but more out of gratitude that I can still do it and possibly a deep understanding that life is for prolonging. I stick to my daily ritual of swimming because I value the ability to keep going. The comment from the man on the train makes more sense now than ever. Another way of looking at it is this:

'It's not how you start out,' said Zig Ziggler, the motivation guru, 'it is how you finish.'

And I am still in the process of finishing: a kind of work in progress philosophy. Long may it continue.

We are all students of life and therefore all practising the work in progress. Belief is not a bad habit to cultivate. To keep going is to keep learning and if there is one lesson that I have learned when writing this book it is that being conscientious brings its own rewards. No-one knows what extends our lifespan, perhaps it is just keeping going.

The Longevity Programme started over ninety years ago with 1500 children being tested, monitored and tracked from childhood to retirement. Howard Friedman and Leslie Martin, two scientists who became involved over the years, have driven the programme to its present conclusions. One of those conclusions is that it is not food that is the answer to a longer life or even activity, but how we interact with others.

Friedman and Martin call this 'consciousness' and that is about nurturing a sense of conscious behaviour. This is nowhere more evident than in the Fitness League. They, like John Higson and Derek Craynor and so many others who I have studied in this book, have a huge ability to be absorbed in what they are doing, so much so that I now believe that what they have mentally is the physical ingredient that keeps them going till the end.

THE EUREKA MOMENT

One of the great advantages of working with all of these people is that I learn so much from them each time we meet.

Sometimes it is just something that comes out of the blue, other times it is something that I learn over time and other times it is a comment or just one line that seems innocuous at the time but then explodes into the conscious mind and you think Eureka!

This happened last on November 10th when Brenda and myself called to see the ladies at St Osmund's in Bolton. We called because I needed to start taking photographs in readiness for this book.

We arrived at about midday. The idea was that I just needed to know who did or did not wish to have their photographs taken. On arriving I saw that they were in the middle of a routine and Ann Hunt was delivering the class to the music of Sam Smith. It was a déjà vu moment because I remember my first visit and Ann was delivering then to Heather Small's 'Looking on up'. This time, however, I noticed something different which brought back memories of meeting and interviewing the ladies.

Lynn Briggs had said in June, 'There is a sense of history with the Fitness League.' Six months on from that interview, I would learn just what she meant and this had nothing to do with the Fitness League and more to do with what happened in 1980 and I not only understood what Lynn meant with history but what it meant to me, this book and Ann Hunt's leadership in the class on the 9th November 2016.

I knew that there was something that I was missing on my early visits to the church hall at St Osmund's. I remember saying to Ann that the class had some kind of connection but I really didn't know what. It was almost like telepathy. It was as though everyone was communicating without a word being spoken.

When Brenda and I entered the hall, Ann had just finished a sequence and was about to start another. The voice of Sam

Smith filled the room and Ann started a rather complicated choreographed routine. All the ladies followed Ann meticulously, every movement perfectly timed, a gentle rhythm with everyone perfectly in tune with Ann and the music. I was immediately thrown back in time to 1980 and the film Fame. The music then could easily have fitted Ann's version of the choreography and for that one brief moment I has the past, the present and the future title for this book. Thirty-seven years later the young people, the cast of the film, would be about the age of the class here at St Osmund's Church in Bolton: three thousand miles across the Atlantic, another time, another place, another group of people, but somehow merging together, a fusion of sound, movement, euphoria, a sense of history and a blend of the present. I knew then that not only did I have my title for this book, but I knew what Lynn Briggs meant with a feeling of history. It was uncanny and that word again, telepathy, came to mind. The harmony, the blend of activity, everyone sharing the moment and what Friedman and Martin would call consciousness.

ASPIRE TO INSPIRE

Immediately after I completed the Boston Marathon, Brenda and I flew to Medford in Southern Oregon. Bill and Judy Pearl's home overlooked the rolling timber-covered mountains and it was this picturesque scene that Bill and I were sharing on a warm sunny morning in the early spring of 1980, renewing our long friendship.

Bill Pearl epitomises success. A Native American, he comes from humble beginnings. At twelve years of age, Bill delivered papers to homes that are probably akin to the council estates in the UK. Bill Pearl's visit to our very humble gym in Bank Street, Bolton in 1969 was a milestone for Bill Stevenson and

I, all those years ago. That was the year that Bill Pearl won the Mr Universe for the fourth time and the guys at our club were both excited and in awe of this icon of world bodybuilding.

It was then that I learned of Bill's background. Being a paper boy on the reservation was the start of his career. One day he spotted an old car in the back yard of a home he was delivering papers to. On asking about the car, the owner agreed to sell it and out of his paper round money Bill Pearl bought the 1924 Ford Model T that would start his collection.

He was already successful when he visited us in 1969: not only was he a huge success as a bodybuilder, but he was a gym owner in the posh area of Los Angeles, Pasadena. His car collection by then was up to twenty-four including two other Ford Model Ts. He also had a thriving mail order company selling protein, vitamin and mineral supplements and he had just started to write his first book Keys to the Inner Universe. Not bad for a Native American born on the reservation.

With all this success, one would wonder why he would visit our rather grotty little gym in a rather scruffy area of Bolton, but he did. This was at a time when the gyms in the UK were still dismal. We had patched up a building to make it look better but it was impossible to make it look nice. We spent hours constantly repainting and renovating and were finding it really difficult to just stay open, yet here we had this very successful bodybuilder and entrepreneur doing nothing but praise our extremely humble attempts at opening a professional health club.

Bill Pearl spent over four hours with us chewing the fat, having a laugh and talking to members and friends who had all come to our gym to meet the mega-star. Bill never saw the flaky paintwork, the damp patch on the ceiling and he never mentioned how basic the equipment was and how it really should be better. All that Bill Pearl could see was the effort that had gone into making a bad property look good. It would have been so easy to say that we needed to do something better with equipment or offer advice on how we structured the programmes, or tell us to move to better and bigger premises. None of that was said, just some subtle advice and the final words just before he left:

'I think you guys are going to make it.'

It was those words that inspired us to do just that. It would have been so easy to have called it a day in 1969. We had given everything to create a business out of the gym. There would have been no shame, no sense of failure. There might have been people who would have scoffed, who would have been glad even, to see a dream disappear but it was that one sentence that reached down into the gut and said 'One more try'. That was in September 1969 and by January 1971, we had moved premises and built a health club that was arguably the best in the country but the idea could so easily have come unstuck if we had not heard those few choice words.

Stickability is part of our existence. All of the characters in this book have that quality. Billy Leach fought like hell to survive the grim conditions of the coal mines. Wynne Barber, now in her late nineties, struggled to survive the Second World War, lost her husband and is now in the early stages of dementia yet she still values her time with the Fitness League and a glass of claret with her evening meal and still encourages her daughter, Lynn, to follow her in that part of her life. Setbacks, failures and illnesses happen and our inherited genes prepare us from birth to struggle but those genes also set us up to succeed. Stickiness is the glue that we cultivate to keep going when we know it may mean failure. Like Thomas Edison when searching for the elusive filament for the light bulb:

'I have not failed,' he said, "I have just found two thousand ways of not doing it.'

Ernest Hemmingway wrote the last chapter of his book A Call To Arms twenty- seven times before he thought it was right. Finding a way is indicative of human nature. Helen Keller, blind, deaf and unable to talk found a way to live a full and productive life. J K Rowling sent her manuscript to twenty seven publishers before her first Harry Potter book was accepted; one publisher telling her that the book was hopeless and she needed to take some writing lessons. Emmeline Pankhurst never gave up believing that women should be equal and have the right to vote. The list is endless: Gandhi, Mandela, Martin Luther King, Rosa Parks, Margaret Thatcher, Theresa May, Angela Merkel, Cleopatra, Winston Churchill, Steve Jobs, Eva Peron, Joan of Arc and Mother Teresa all found a way and built a better life for themselves and for others. From Florence Nightingale to Coco Chanel, from the greatest equal rights activist of all time Shivaji Bhonsle, the Hindu leader to Jesus Christ, stickability is the substance of greatness.

NEVER GIVE UP

Joe Heathcote came from a mining family. The average age of his forbears was fifty-two. Poverty, ignorance, social inequality and the lack of opportunity were probably the causes of his situation. Joe broke the rules: a professional fight in his early life should have left him punch drunk or with dementia but it didn't. A broken back when aged thirty-four should have left him jobless for life but it didn't. A severe heart attack at the age of fifty-eight, leaving him with angina, should have seen him off but it didn't. Poverty and the lack of any recognised skills should have had him following in his forbears' footsteps and seen him dead long before his sixtieth birthday, but he lived until four weeks before his ninety-seventh birthday. Joe Heathcote never gave up on life. Life gave up on Joe.

As an example of all the great people in the world past or present, I need to look no further than my Dad. I suspect that all of my family today would have the same opinion if asked. I think that all of us, every woman or every child, would have no reason to look any further than their friends and family. We are surrounded by inspiration. We are blessed with people we know who lift our hearts, feed us with positives, give us joy and fill our lives with love. All we have to do us look, shift gear into drive and plan to go forward instead of in reverse.

NEVER GIVE UP

There are many interpretations of a speech that Winston Churchill gave to the students of his old school, Harrow. It really matters not what was said except that the words inspired the audience. The story goes that in 1941 he was invited to address the pupils. The whole speech was two pages long and somewhere in the middle Churchill delivered these immortal words:

'Never give in. Never give in. Never, never, never, never give in.'

These words of the man whom many believe was Britain's greatest Briton, were just one of his comments out of so many for those who looked to lift their spirits in their times of need.

At times we all need some form of inspiration. I know that over the years I have sought something to lift the sagging spirits, some motivation, something that would release the adrenalin or get the taste buds of my brain to galvanise the body into action. Hormones and particularly neurotransmitters that release dopamine can kick start a new wave of energy and enthusiasm. Not everything in life is about sudden bursts or the quick reaction. In fact, it is just about the opposite and to realise that, I had to go back to what the ladies had said on my first visit to the Fitness League and that one word that changed my way of thinking.

SUSTAINABILITY: THE ANSWER?

It must be in the blood because after sixty odd years of working out I still keep track of how the fitness industry is progressing. The industry as a whole is not very good at holding on to customers: the average club in the country and in America will show figures of less than fifty percent retention. Many clubs will show far less than that with a loss of up to eighty or ninety per cent. This is a staggering statistic when you think of the appalling figures for obesity and diabetes and the colossal amount of money spent on medicine. All that, plus having a National Health Service that is desperately near collapse and doctors threatening strikes. How we rectify this is an issue that the country needs to sort but in truth we are no nearer to a solution than we have ever been. Yet the answer is really quite simple and part of that answer might just come from a ninety-six year study on longevity.

Doctors Howard S Friedman and Leslie R Martin are both flying the flag for this extremely worthwhile project. Now this is not a book about longevity but is a book about living until you die and both of these ways of life come together in some way. For one thing we do agree that it's not about diet or exercise, though both have a part to play. We also agree that community (tribe) plays a huge part and we also agree that having a good disposition or attitude of mind is a major factor. For that, see our case studies and look at the examples of Billy Leach, Sylvia Faucitt, Derek Craynor and all our 'girls' at the Fitness League. There is so much in common between these people and the Longevity Programme that at times it's hard to separate them.

What we can all learn from Friedman and Martin is that sociability is one of the key issues in finding the secrets to eternal youth. People need people and they need to feel that they matter and are valued and that the people around them are like them. In Friedman's studies they used selected students. These students considered themselves special and dubbed themselves 'Terman's Termites' after the originator of the programme, Lewis Terman, a psychologist at Stamford University. The Termites feeling that they were part of a group even a special group is described in the study as one of their personality traits.

Fundamental to this study, and to the people of this book, is the fact that all of them value the community spirit and in the health clubs of today that is not just missing but is not even encouraged. This one ingredient can change the dynamic of health club membership: not only will it lead to membership retention but it will keep more people active longer and therefore help them stay healthy and in addition improve their moods and sense of participation and that means stickiness.

All clubs are social clubs. Rotary Clubs, Labour Clubs, Conservative Clubs, rugby, football, cricket, the Lyon's Round Table, the Women's Inner Wheels and the new networking clubs, the engineering institute, golf clubs, bowling, rambling, swimming, triathlon clubs and running clubs. Every one is designed to be a social gathering that encourages participation. The purpose is to keep people together: stickiness.

The Minister for Health should find a way of making health clubs responsible for people's health. What good is it being fit if you're not healthy? What good is it to look good, have big muscles and have the figure of a goddess if you're not healthy? What good is it if clubs sign people up for a year and they leave in three months, or a year or two years? Health is for life. Health needs stickability.

BEING OF A MIND

The other day I met an old member of our club. She is now well into her seventies and was feeling a little sorry for herself because she had just put on eight pounds.

'I have just joined a club and they do Pilates,' she said.

Good, I thought, Pilates is excellent like yoga or any form of class that encourages meditation. All these encourage concentration and what is now being called consciousness, a term used for having a conscious mind. All exercise should serve that purpose: it is very hard to think of anything else if you are absorbed in what you do. Just to do laps in the pool will not absorb you. Just going through a pump class will not absorb you if you don't work hard. Spinning, treadmill, rower or HIIT will not absorb you or take you into a good place if you do not work hard enough to separate your mind from your everyday existence. Working hard and boredom do not go together. Without the concentration of mind you do not get the consciousness. Exercise shuts out the garbage, lifts the spirits, gives the feel-good factor but it will never work unless you work at both the exercise and the stickability.

I didn't say to my friend, the old member, that she would find it hard losing eight pounds with Pilates but if she works at the classes steadily and sticks to the programme what it will do is help to change the mind to help keep the body going. She will then need to develop the good habits and leave the bad habits out if sight. She will also develop an attitude of regularity that becomes ritualistic to get into her zone, the zone that encourages stickiness.

Ed Whitlow finds training a drag, but trains so that he

can compete. Mary McDaid's philosophy is to keep doing the Fitness League so that both sides of the brain are working in addition to the body. Derek Craynor hates the thought of rust and Sylvia Faucitt is always looking for reasons to continue. Sally Floyd in Edinburgh wants her students to keep doing her classes forever, so that she can go on forever too.

I will keep having my coffee and spend as much time doing it as I do swimming, but you see I value my time drinking coffee with friends just as much as I value my swim. That way we will all keep going and all keep sticking to our rituals.

20 – PLACE

What price place? How much does our environment affect our health and well-being? We know that in the past, up until the 1960s, people had major problems with air pollution and industrial waste. We know now that poor living conditions and ignorance of nutrition can affect longevity. We know now that there is a difference geographically in life expectancy. The long living areas of Okinawa, Sardinia and other places like Loma Linda in California, have the availability of more natural food, clean air and unstressful environments. These things obviously have an effect on the quality of life but are they the real answer or is there some other contributory factor?

The latest studies from across the world now show that food and exercise play a less important role in good health and longevity. There seems to be more emphasis on community and the individual's personality in unselfishly mixing with others. Certainly with people like the Fitness League my findings fit these global studies. People like Billy Leach, Dad and other people from the mines, from engineering, from the factories and other contaminated industrial units had no chance. This has now changed and people are now benefiting from that change.

The global studies and my study of a few hundred people in the UK agree. It is not the diet nor is it the activity but where we are mentally, a mentality that gives out, shares a common ground, a genuine interest in others.

'There is no I here,' said Dan Buettner in the mountains of a Blue Zone, and one of the six places on the planet were people live longer. 'It is not the geographical place but where we position our minds that count'.

Every single one of the people who I interviewed with the Fitness League insisted it was the camaraderie, the friendship, the laughter and the 'sharing' of the experience. As soon as they walked through the door of the church hall at St Osmund's Church they stepped into another place. This is happening all over the world, not just with the Fitness League but almost everyone who I met with. Derek Craynor twice a week visits to the gym changed his mentality. Fifty years ago it did the same for Billy Leach. Sylvia Faucitt's ritual of exercise keeps her happy. Mary McDaid in County Wicklow would be in a good place wherever she was. Hamish McPherson is happy in the gym and Sally Floyd in Edinburgh is happy because her ladies will be with her till the day they die. The physical environment is not the issue nor the saviour but the place in your mind is.

Ed Whitlow, the octogenarian superman of running, said that training can be a drag. What makes Ed happy is the competition: he loves to race and when he races he is in a good place regardless of where the race is. What Billy Leach was saying fifty years ago was reiterating these beliefs. Health comes from within. Billy's mantra came from his mind and I guess from his heart. Only the coal miner's cancer could defeat Billy. Attitude of mind is crucial. This not only comes from global studies and the longevity project, but from the mouths of these seventy, eighty and even ninety year old babes. They've got it. By George, they've got it!

Ulrich Inderbinen had the distinction of almost living into three centuries. Born in December 1900, he lived to be 105 years of age. Ulrich climbed the Matterhorn no less than 370 times, the last time at the age of 90.

Inderbinen's early life was extremely hard. At five years of age he was tending to the animals on the smallholding high in the Alps of Switzerland. Food was hard to come by: maize, vegetables and meat when it was available. The Inderbinen family were the last of the Swiss nomads moving around the mountains to catch the seasons and whatever food the seasons brought.

Ulrich's first attempt to climb the iconic mountain was at the age of twenty. He and his two sisters set off one morning, his sisters dressed in ordinary street clothes: long frocks and casual shoes. None of them knew the route to the top, so they followed scratch marks from other climbers' boots to guide them to the summit. It took them four hours to reach the top. Seventy years later he made his final accent and it took him four and a half hours.

He became one of the most prolific mountain guides of all time. He also became a top ski instructor and later a competitor in skiing events across the Alps. His last skiing event was at the age of ninety. Not the easiest man to interview but when pinned down he was found to have a dry sense of humour. On one occasion, he was seen carrying two pairs of large wooden skis. When asked why two sets, he quipped that one set was for him and the other set for his Dad.

Ulrich Inderbinen was a very moderate eater. He ate meat sparingly and cow's milk was very much part of his daily intake. He often said that once he started hiking or climbing he hated to stop, so he took very few rest periods. He would often hike for four or five hours at a time even into his late nineties. His simple fare and his approach to ritualistic exercise, is in keeping with most of our people in this book. His tough upbringing and work ethic is reminiscent of the likes of Billy Leach, Dad, Hamish McPherson and Derek Craynor, and ninety-five year old John Higson. The common denominator in all of these people is their attitude to life: no fuss, no excuses; we do it because we like it. And they hated it when they missed.

There is no consistency in the exterior environment of all of these people. For decades, researchers and academic instructors have continually championed two things that dictate longevity: diet and location. The longevity project, however, refutes both of these theories at least in part, with attitude being the most prominent factor and quality and persistence being key. Inderbinen and our current batch of people demonstrated their habits of not giving up. This is obvious with Sylvia Faucitt, Ann Hunt and Lynn Ward and their mothers: sticking with it not for just one generation but for two. History, tradition and reliability are important as is the place in our minds that says I want to do this.

This book is not about living to be a hundred or more but it is about having the presence of mind to change if we need to. One of the big features of the longevity project is how divorce impacts on longevity, as do drug abuse and smoking. Stay active, sleep well, don't gain weight and be careful with what you eat. In other words eliminate the grotty things in life and start introducing the better things. There are some things however that we cannot change, like being born in or after the industrial revolution, or our history of poverty or being born into families that disregard healthy habits or don't cultivate good habits. Perhaps when Lynn Ward said that history was a quality that she admired and a reason why she's still involved with the Fitness League, she was more perceptive than I thought at the time.

The seeds were planted with the words of Derek Craynor's grandmother. She said 'If you rest you rust' and that single line steered Derek to a better way of life. Or Sylvia Faucitt's 'reasons rather than excuses'. To me it is not luck or coincidence that John Higson's prophesy of living to be a hundred came true, but more a question of attitude. Dad would say to me 'Just keep going'. He did this with words but he also set a personal example. 'Lets just do one length' when the water was freezing, and no-one else would swim, was probably the best example of all: still doing something, failing sometimes.

Inferno, hell, abyss, grave, misery and wretchedness are all words that we associate with Hell. My first and only trip into the bowels of the earth was to the Brackley Colliery in 1949, a school trip to experience the working life of the miner. 'Hell on earth' was the thought that filled my mind. Total blackness, white teeth and eyes and the low glimmer of the miner's lamp. The near naked men clad in boots, underpants and a helmet. Nothing showing of the pale white flesh, not even an inch showing through the fine, translucent gossamer of black dust. Voices, teeth and eyes the only signs of human existence, as at fourteen years of age I crouched low beneath a ledge called the coal face.

Sixty-six years later, the closing of the last deep coal mine in Britain would attract the press, television and thousands of people to watch the end of an era. Crowds lined the streets of nearby Knottingley in West Yorkshire, to watch as the pitmen walked the mile from the pit to the miners' social club. Memories came flooding back to me, not from the brief time of my solitary visit to a mine, but from my father's years spent a thousand or two thousand feet below and the hundred of stories that Dad related to me about a time over seventy years ago. Not a place to be in body or mind. Clearly conditions are better now. A vast change brought about by government legislation, health and safety and the constant pressure from unions, activists and campaigners who wanted a safer workface for the warriors of the deep. There seems to be no limit to the survival instincts of the human mind and body. The horrors of the mines were unfolded to me as Dad relived them so many times. Coal blasted like shrapnel, bodies maimed, limbs lost, death: a daily risk, an accepted consequence of a desperate need to provide food, clothing and shelter for families. A time and place and an unyielding environment that gave so little back except life itself and maybe pride of place.

CULTURE

Visionaries see the end first; others just see the problem. Mary Bagot Stack saw a better place for women through the realms of exercise. Emily Pankhurst and her suffragettes had sacrificed life and limb so that women could hold their place in society. Mary Bagot Stack was a simple extension of what the suffragettes has achieved. In the early days of 1932 when Stack created her vision, she would not have known that she was forming a culture and a mindset that would impact on students nearly a hundred years in the future. Out of her philosophy, women would form exercise classes across the world. Hundreds of thousands of women would join the Fitness League, each of them shaping a culture of belonging.

When I started the research into the League almost a year ago, Lynn Ward spoke with great affection about loyalty, history and feeling secure among her friends. Since then Lynn was diagnosed with breast cancer and has undergone surgery.

'I can't wait,' she said, 'to get back and take my place, third from the back and on the left, we are like squaddies. I am looking forward to getting my mojo back.'

Lynn takes part in other classes elsewhere.

'I am missed at the other classes, but not like the Fitness League. You see,' she said, 'I'm going back to family.'

I wonder if Mary Bagot Stack had seen that bond and the feeling of security, comfort, pride and belonging. Lynn Ward like Sylvia Faucitt and all her colleagues at the Fitness League know that they have something special in that one and a half hour exercise class in that small church hall in Bolton. It is not just a group of women exercising to music: it is a belief, a regime and a culture that spreads across the world. I didn't see that a year ago but I do now.

PEOPLE AND PLACES

I spent just two years with Her Majesty's Forces and was uncomfortable both physically and mentally. I knew then that I wasn't made to be a soldier but it didn't stop me appreciating the value. Like a lot of others I could not wait for demob. Now sixty years on I realise just how important it was in the provision of a rounded life. Those two years were a blur. Basic training, then the move to the Para Regiment, a year of active service in Cyprus, EOKA, General Grivas, Archbishop Makarios, weapon training, parachute jumping, patrols in the mountains, a year under canvas and a camaraderie equal to the Fitness League, the coal miners and the forty years of looking after our customers at Bolton Health Studios. Now at eighty one years of age I am what is called an ambassador for the fitness industry. People have come and gone, events have faded into the past: the London Palladium, the Scala Theatre, the new and old Victoria Palace; John Paul Getty, Arnold Schwarzenegger, Bill Pearl, Oscar Heidenstam, Jonah Barrington, Des Drummond, Sebastian Coe, the first London Marathon, Boston, Roger Boubon, Beverley Hills, Prince Charles and Sammy Davies Junior. People, places, a different time, a different place and a different way of thinking.

FINDING YOUR PLACE

Ed Whitlock loves to compete, so each day he runs around Toronto's Central Cemetery and hacks out the miles. Lynn Ward is now over her cancer and can't wait to get back to her place at the Fitness League. Tony Ford at 84 will play his ten games a week at the various bowling clubs near to his home. Today, tomorrow and every day I will eat up the laps in the pool so that I can meet the challenge of Windermere. Hamish McPherson at nearly 90 is finding it hard to workout at the gym but wouldn't miss out for the world. Billy Leach used to make his trips to the Harriers because he loved the camaraderie and they let him vent his philosophy. Bill and Judy Pearl get up 'at 4 am to workout in the gym because it is so much worse not to. These and all the people in this book have found a place in their minds to feel satisfied with what they do and why they do it.

'It's not doing what you like,' said Dad, 'But liking what you do.'

Tony Ford, on the death of his wife found his salvation in crown green bowling. 'I didn't take to it straight away,' he said, 'but after a few games I couldn't stop. I now play every day and even go on bowling holidays.

Sylvia Faucitt fell downstairs and broke her neck, then found a future through exercise. Dad's broken back led to a life of lifting weights, swimming and long walks.

There are millions out there in the world who have turned their lives around through exercise. Some have turned to religion; some to friends. The band of mothers who lost their sons in Afghanistan turned to each other and helped the survivors. All got out of this place and started a new life with new goals and new ambitions.

In the words of the lead singer in the Animals, Eric Burdon: 'We gotta get out of this place, if it's the last thing we ever do, cos girl there's a better life for me and for you.' Make the move.

PLACE

The word fun was always associated with vaudeville, the theatre, the circus or the pleasure parks at holiday resorts.

Now it's fun to exercise, work out at gyms, do fun runs for twenty-six miles. It's fun to do spinning classes, aerobics and even high intensity interval training, but training and fun don't really gel. Ask Chris Hoy or Bradley Wiggins, or Mo Farah when he is spewing up when taking himself to V^O2 max for too long. There is a difference between training and just doing exercise. A fun run is only fun until you start punishing your body to get that extra inch or that extra ounce of energy, or that extra few seconds out of a race.

Extending our limits is not fun: it's serious business. Taxing ourselves to our limits to the extent of collapse is taking our body and mind beyond our comfort zones. Being serious is the opposite of fun. Training is doing it when you don't want to. Training is discipline and training and discipline have nothing to do with fun. Not every training session takes us to our limits, it is then that there is time for some fun but inevitably the fun stops.

Ask Bradley Wiggins if his training is fun and he will probably tell you to go away. Training at top level is brutal. Brutal and fun don't mix.

HIGH INTENSITY INTERVAL TRAINING AND PAIN

It is now nearly forty years since I made the attempt to run from John O'Groats to Lands End. There are a number of different routes to this mammoth task, with the least mileage being about seven hundred and fifty miles. There was a rather vague record for this and the distance had allegedly been covered in ten days. This meant that I had to cover approximately eighty miles a day.

I made the mistake of changing my running shoes from Reebok to New Balance the day before setting out on my epic run. Both Reebok and New Balance are excellent shoes, but do have certain characteristics that differentiate the foot-plant and in particular the lifting of the heel on the trailing leg. In other words the heel on the New Balance is different to the one on the Reebok shoe.

In ordinary training or competition this would have little effect, but if the shoes need to carry me for seventy or eighty miles a day then this minor difference is greatly magnified. Right from the first day and a few thousand strides into the first eighty miles, the Achilles tendon on my left leg began to complain. Fatigue was already setting in and I had only just started.

Pain is defined as an unpleasant subjective experience whose purpose is to motivate you to do something; usually to protect body parts that the brain thinks are damaged. If you feel pain it thinks the body is under threat and the brain thinks it has to do something about it.

Pain is a survival mechanism. Pain is an output of the brain. It's telling you to lower your intensity and by the time I had reached day two, the brain had given up.

I ran on automatic pilot for eight days averaging seventy miles a day. For all of those eight days I was battling with the survival mechanism that was telling me to stop, and on the eighth day I did. Nearly four decades later I still feel that pain. This time it is the emotional feeling of 'what if?' What if I had settled for a lower mileage? What if I hadn't changed my shoes? What if I had training less intensely?

What that painful experience did do was to teach me about the pitfalls of overdoing and over use and it taught me in, no uncertain terms, that we have to respect what the brain is telling us to do.

The new wave of HIIT is good but only if we listen and respond to the pitfalls of constant activity and pace ourselves accordingly.

I know that I have explained V^{O}2 Max in another part of the book, but let me reiterate about the downside of HIIT. High Intensity means taking your pulse rate to near maximum. We measure this by deducting our age from 220. So if you are 50 years of age your maximum pulse rate is 170. High Intensity means keeping your pulse rate for a given number of seconds (intensity) before resting for a given number of seconds (interval).

Pain is good. Pain is the catalyst that releases the endorphins that make us feel good. One of these endorphins is called dopamine. This is released when we reach our limit of 170 beats of the pulse if you are 50. This is sometimes called 'pumped'. We get 'pumped up' by exertion (HIIT). This is a process and it is regulated by three main neurotransmitters: serotonin, norepinephrine; and dopamine. All this is good not just for the body but for the brain as well but there is a balance and the balance is to regulate the exercise to acceptable levels.

Finding the balance is dependent on exercise, our background and our DNA. Are we as individuals deigned for intensity? Are we explosive by nature? Do we have the right balance of fast twitch fibres and slow twitch fibres? Intensive exercise asks a lot of questions and those questions become more acute when we get older. Age and intensity are like oil and water; they are very difficult to mix.

High Intensity Interval Training (HIIT) is good but less good with age. The amount of training in the red (high intensity) for trained athletes is just 5% or in simple terms, five minutes in every hour. That is for trained athletes, not the regular keep-fitter. Much of that calculation is based on background, history, length of time training and the nature of the sport or activity. Endurance athletes find it difficult to go to the extreme. Ed Whitlock and Derek Craynor both extremely fit, shy away from intensity. I do ten miles a week in the water but find it hard to go into oxygen debt (maximum pulse rate): that is probably my brain telling me not to go into that intensity pain area, just another factor to consider when trying HIIT.

Exercise and physical activity puts you into a place that can ether be pleasant or painful. It can leave us hot or it can leave us cold, exhilarated or tired, on top of the world or down in the dumps, with a feeling of buoyancy or that sinking feeling. Listen to your brain.

21 – PRIDE

One of the proudest moments of my working life was when Jonah Barrington came to our club in Bolton. This was a legend of world squash, six times world champion and a man reckoned to be the fittest man in the world. Jonah came, not for money or publicity, nor even to do us a favour but just because he wanted to see what we were doing with our gym.

You will notice that I said one of the proudest moments of my working life. Pride in one's family can never be measured against anything else. The proudest moments are always in seeing our children come into the world, seeing them grow and flourish, and then seeing them have children of their own. There is nothing that can beat seeing your grandchild taking their place in the world. Becoming a Grandma and Granddad is one of the most emotional times of anyone's life. To see the succession, the continuation and the future is a feeling that is unsurpassed and to still be around when that third generation comes along, well, pride is part of our DNA and there is nothing more significant in life than life itself.

Jonah's visit would start a friendship that would go on for years, with only miles and circumstances separating the bond. Our business in the seventies and eighties was totally dependent on making people aware of what we were trying to do. This was at a time when there was no awareness of a profession that kept people fit. I remember being approached by Yellow Pages: did we want to be entered into a telephone directory? That year 1969, there was not one single entry for gyms, let alone health clubs or studios. A few years after our first entry in the directory, Jonah Barrington asked if he could visit our new business, a gym that had dared to gamble on the game of squash. We were very proud of what we had achieved: squash courts alongside beauty therapy and a crèche for kids. No one was doing this and the great man himself was hailing our vision.

The chest swells, they eyes glisten and the blood surges through the brain. Pride inspires children and adults alike. Watching the children and the grandchildren on the playing fields of sport gave us more pleasure than we cared to admit. It's not the winning but the taking part that counts. The saying is never more true when seeing your children grow up.

Pride, however, goes much deeper than the rush of blood to the head. Pride can soon become arrogance when the feeling of satisfaction turns to superiority. No one I know, however, didn't feel proud when graduating from college with a degree, dressed in cap and gown or sitting there having a photo taken on the day that celebrates an achievement. No one who has even an ounce of patriotism would not be proud of our athletes who competed in the Olympic Games. Everyone who saw Andy Murray play tennis experienced some pleasure in seeing him become world champion. The human being is the only animal on this planet that feels emotion for others. We can feel good about ourselves and we can feel good for others. We can feel good about ourselves because we feel good for others.

Heather Small's 'Proud' is not just motivation, but it has stirred the blood of many.

'What have you done today that makes you feel proud?'

The words lifted the hearts of millions at the 2012 Olympic Games; each and every one of us so proud of the athletes who represented us. They in turn strove to win so that we could be proud of them. The power of pride is a rare ingredient in our make up when used properly. Pride, on the other hand can be destructive self-obsession, arrogance or an unenviable feeling of superiority. Pride, along with greed, avarice, gluttony, envy, lust, and sloth, make up the seven deadly sins, the opposites being humility, kindness, abstinence, chastity, patience, diligence and liberty.

There is nothing wrong with the feel-good factor. We feel good about losing those few inches, dropping a dress size, still being active into old age. I felt good about myself when interviewing Derek Craynor and Ann Hunt at the Fitness's League. I felt proud to have known Billy Leach. The interviews with Mary McDaid, Lynn Ward and John Higson made my heart soar, put a skip in my step and polished my ego, just because I shared their lives even if it was only for those moments. There is no better feeling than being part of something shared and feeling a pride in others.

Oscar Heidenstam was a former soldier: on his demob he worked in physical culture which we now call the fitness industry. Oscar formed an organisation called the National Amateur Bodybuilders Association (NABBA). He later took that to a new level and organised the Mr Universe competition. This organisation grew and both NABBA and the Mr Universe enjoyed world fame. Both attracted hundreds of thousands of people who wanted to be part of this tribe called 'bodybuilders'. People from almost every country in the world would make the journey to London to watch for over fifty years. People from the little back street gyms of Porto Rica to the Australian outback, from Bangladesh to Palm Springs, from Ireland to Hawaii and from Washington DC to Brussels. They would all come to London and Oscar would pay homage to these young people and put them onto the greatest stages in the world: the Scala Theatre, the Old Victoria Palace, the New Victoria Palace and the London Palladium. The West End of London hosted kids from the back street gyms who trained with barbells and dumbbells, black iron weights, producing the best bodybuilders in the world.

Arnold Schwarzenegger, Sean Connery (who would later become James Bond), and Steve Reeves who would portray Hercules in Hollywood: these were names that were only known in the world of bodybuilding but were icons to the millions of fans across the world. Oscar made bodybuilding respectful when it was still hidden away in cellars, school halls, rooms above pubs, storage units, some old mill or garage or the back yard of a terraced house. Now, sixty or seventy years on, we have health clubs across the world, part of a multi-billion dollar industry. Billions are spent on watches, protein drinks, clothing, shoes, and all the accessories that didn't exist in the seventies and eighties. Oscar brought respectability to people who were only seen as superficial characters, who posed and just looked good to the uncritical eye. Now we cannot open a paper, read a magazine or watch a film without someone's pecs being on display. Rugby and football players and all kind of Olympians are admired not just for their skills, but for their abs, cuts and well-proportioned bodies. Jessica Ennis, Camila Giorgi, the Italian tennis star, Ellen Hoog, the Dutch hockey player and Meghan Hardin, a female pro-athlete with multiple skills and also a beautiful model, tennis's Williams sisters, Whitney Miller, the top wake surfer and long jumper, and Voula Papachristou all demonstrate muscle, skill, beauty and agility. Oscar Heidenstam started that trend over seventy years ago by putting physical excellence onto the greatest platforms in the world. Who could not be proud of knowing this bodybuilder, writer, innovator and pioneer.

UNDERSTANDING

Heidi Boyle is seventy-six years old and swims daily. Her daily ritual is about sixty lengths of a pool thirty metres long. In overall terms Heidi swims approximately one mile five days a week. She hardly every mentions this fact to anyone but if you asked if she was proud of this, she would undoubtedly say 'Yes'. Who would not be proud of doing a daily swim of a mile at 76?

Sue Catterall is sixty-three years of age and has been a keen marathon runner for nearly thirty years. Two years ago, she decided to learn how to swim properly. Now she swims three to four times a week and this year she swam the Great North Swim in Lake Windermere, a distance of one mile. This year it is her intention to do the two mile event and then next year the 5K, all in open water.

We now have a phenomenon of 'old' people who work out. They hike, bike, swim, lift weights, play tennis, golf, bowls, do spin classes, body attack, aerobics, palates, yoga, and train with free weights. If you asked them if they did it to impress they would be mortified. They do it because they want a better life, a fuller life, a life that is more fulfilling, a life with goals, aspirations, and a life that is socially involved with people because they want to. The critics could say that it is self-admiration, narcissistic or a way of feeling superior over others. All of these people, both women and men cultivate a sense of pride. Pride in their own efforts, pride in their own achievements, and pride in their own self esteem.

Bill Pearl, my mate from Oregon in the USA, once said that his priority was to look after himself so that he could look after others. How can I look after the people who rely on me if I am not in a fit state of mind and body? How can I look after others? Yes, there are the egotistical types but once you reach a certain age in life you learn to understand that this life does not go on forever. Self-cultivation is not just about pride, but about survival.

For years I have stood on speaking platforms at home and abroad: at Wembley, the National Exhibition Centre in

Birmingham, Blackpool, Brighton and so many of the smaller venues. Most of my talks were on marketing, customer service, motivation and sales. Sharing my knowledge was never a question of ego. Just standing up in front of your peers can be a nerve-wracking experience. I learned a long time ago that public speaking was an essential part of a business that relied on projecting the advantages of the product. Businesses call this marketing; the church calls it preaching. I cannot yet come to terms with the fact that marketing and sales are looked upon with some suspicion. Preaching and sermonising are the words of the church and marketing and sales are the words that arouse suspicion. There is somehow a feeling of something not right with the ways of business as opposed to virtue, the language of religion. I am proud that I was asked to speak at the National Conference Centre: it was always a challenge to hold an audience. Yes, it massaged my ego but at the same time it was appreciated by the audience, it was valued. Expertise is peculiar: it has a unique quality of enriching those who receive it, without diminishing those who give it away. Public speaking gives and receives. The speaker gives his knowledge away and the audience receives that gift with applause and appreciation.

One of the great things in life for me has been to listen and learn from great speakers. I have travelled this world and relished and wallowed in the knowledge of others. I felt proud to stand up and spread the word on the subjects of my talks. Only a few years ago, I was asked to speak to young people who were contemplating going into business. This was a government programme to promote entrepreneurship and to get people into self-employment. I travelled throughout the region delivering talks on making the next step, the giant leap into business. To know that you have done a good job and to have an audience respond is a great feeling. I am still proud of that sensation, a feeling that you are acknowledged for what you know, but more importantly for how you transfer that knowledge to others. Pride is perhaps a bit egotistical but a small price for enriching others.

This year I will once more be invited to officiate at the National Fitness Awards, a sort of Oscars or BAFTA event. This year my role will be the diplomat. I am sensing that there is a feeling that I am slowing down and I am, but isn't it good to be wanted, to be valued, to think that someone out there will feel better for your presence? Does that not stir the blood just a little or make me feel just a little proud.

BE PROUD OF WHO YOU ARE

Where would the world be without pride? How would we survive without our heroes? Why is it considered that pride is a sin? What would become of us without something to aim for, someone to admire, or a goal to boost our feeling of self?

Sir Edmund Hillary conquered the highest summit. Amelia Earhart flew across the Atlantic. Roger Bannister ran the four minute mile. I felt so proud when Jessica Ennis won gold then we had Victoria Pendleton in cycling and what about Bradley Wiggins and Jason Kenny? I would dare anyone to dent my pride in the fourth generation, namely our great-grand-daughter Sophia Rose Thorpe. Of course, pride is important, pride is good not evil and pride lifts our spirits, flushes our cheeks and lifts our head up high.

EUPHORIA

Last year was my sixth year at the National Fitness Awards. The Awards are organised by Script Media, a subsidiary of Workout Magazine, and by many other companies that come under the umbrella of the Acredula Group. My first visit to this hugely impressive event was in 2011 when I was awarded the prestigious Lifetime Achievement Award. This was to be my third Lifetime Achievement Award and each time I feel nothing but pride that other people think me worthy of their judgement. This award started another chain of events that saw me once more judging other people to be in line for similar awards.

This year in Leicester, eight hundred people turned out to celebrate other people winning the various categories for this national event. There were awards for the Best Health Club, Best Budget Club, Best Rehabilitation Centre, Best Local Authority Fitness Centre: twenty-two awards in all with eight hundred people clapping, whistling, punching the air, or just wallowing in the euphoria and adrenalin of the occasion. All proud for their colleagues, the reward and the recognition.

'Wouldn't it be nice,' someone said, 'to have fame without having attention but a short burst of attraction can only be good for the soul?'

It was Voltaire who said 'We are rarely proud when we are alone.'

No one was alone at the Fitness Awards. Reward and recognition is good for our egos and should be accepted with a large degree of humility..

I don't know if it's by accident or by some inherent design, but I have not been witness often to the claim that pride is a vice and not a virtue. Many years ago I was involved yet again in the world of judging. This time it was at the Mr Universe competition in London. The late Oscar Heidenstam was the man who created a great event that attracted people from all over the world to compete for the best physique on the planet. To be a judge at this very prestigious show was a very proud time in my career. Why ask me? Why choose me to judge these people from India, Australia, America; competitors from all over Europe, South Africa, Porta Rica, Venezuela, Ecuador and just about anywhere on the planet? It was the equivalent of world soccer or rugby, of Wimbledon and, for those young competitors, the chance to get on stage at the London Palladium, the Victoria Palace or the Scala Theatre was just astonishing. Young men out of the back street gyms mostly with no luxury or even basic facilities for washing, or showering facilities were going from one extreme to the other. Their pride could only be matched by their humility. I met them, got to know them and shared their stories, their time and I even dined with them. Just ordinary people from ordinary homes, ordinary working class people who had no reservations about showing their pride, win or lose, in just being part of the bigger picture, the organisation that embraced their sport. How can anyone deny their pride of place in that?

We do things because we want to do things. We continue to do things because we deserve something out of what we do, then there comes a point where we either let go or it becomes part of our own culture, our character, and the thing, whatever it is, becomes us. There are millions of people who dedicate themselves to charities, to sport, or to the benefit of others. Every community in the world has someone who embraces a cause or a philosophy, a dream, a mission, a charity, or a belief. They aspire to inspire and by doing their thing they attract the admiration and the respect of people around them and for that they should be proud. Those who think that that is wrong, that pride is a sin should look no further than themselves and ask themselves where they stand in this place they call the world.

I, like many of my contemporaries, would like to turn the clock back, to put right what I now know to be wrong such as a word or casual remark, to change a direction or decision or to just listen instead of just talking. Serendipity is fine in retrospect. Would I have gone away, knowing that Dad was going to die? What would I have said, done or changed? In all probability nothing, because that is life, except maybe something could have been better.

It was during one of those moments that I thought of the man who changed bodybuilding. Oscar, a former professional soldier, started a movement called the National Amateur Bodybuilding Association and by doing that changed the world for millions of people. I was proud to be part of that even though it was only a small part. I was proud to have known Oscar. I was proud to have met the thousands who were involved. I was proud that I met Bill Pearl and forged a friendship.

My life and the people around me were all part of that period in our lives that enriched us and for that reason we should be proud of those little things that provide us with the feel-good factor.

The brain's reward system, i.e. the hypothalamus, is discussed in the chapter on Mind. The main component of the brain's reward system is a neural pathway call the mesolimbic pathway. This system produces the neurotransmitter dopamine, the substance that elevates our senses and gives us that pumped-up feeling. Good news, praise from others, reaching a goal, scoring a goal, or just receiving a pat on the back, can all activate the 500,000 dopamine producing neurons that give our ego a boost.

THE WOW FACTOR

Over a ten year period I worked with a number of companies installing a customer care philosophy. In every single case, the philosophy revolves around a reward and recognition programme. What we had to accomplish was the staff's approach to customer care. Because of my background in running gyms and health clubs I was already more than halfway there in knowing what the customer wanted and in particular how they felt about our product. In order to make this work we first had to install a sense of pride in the staff. The reward and recognition programme had to motivate both the customer and the staff. We called this The Moments of Magic Programme.

The object of the exercise was to send the customer away punching the air with delight. Just as important was the feeling from the staff that they too wanted to punch the air because they made it happen for the customer. The catalyst for this was to let the staff come up with the ideas that enthused the customer. We called this 'the licence to thrill'. We made it fun. Fun for the staff. Fun for the customer. The results of this initiative were extraordinary. We would see unbelievable 'moment of magic'. The staff would learn to entertain them, turn moments of misery into moments of magic and they would learn that there were moments of truth. Letting these people create these moments would install a sense of pride, a sense of accomplishment and a sense of satisfaction.

On one of many occasions a young employee won the employee of the month award. Her reward was the recognition of her peers, another was recognition from her employer and another recognition from the customer; but the real twist in this was the recognition from her family. This recognition came when she took the small Oscar-like trophy home and her Dad, on seeing it broke down in tears. His little daughter had been recognised above all the other members of staff to be the best and that little trophy still stands over the fireplace ten years after it was won. What price the pride in that!

Striving to achieve is a natural function of the human brain, part of that mind set that we covered earlier in the book. We are born to achieve and to survive: without that compulsion the human race would have ceased to exist more than a million years ago. The mechanism of the brain functions through emotion, and emotion fires up the blood and we feel good about ourselves. Setting ourselves targets is not just about ego, but about surviving everything that life can throw at us. The challenge to just exist is just as vital today as it was in the times of our ancestors. The evolution of the species today is different from a million years ago but no less threatening than it was then. We have a greater access to knowledge today than in ancient times, we live longer and we are healthier. We have medicine and experience. We have greater comforts and the day to day fight for survival is different, but is still there. The fight today is not physical, but mental, the fight today is about mental capacity in old age and the challenge is one of sanity with the oncoming war with dementia. It is one thing to live to be a hundred and another to know that you are a hundred.

22 – FAT

Fat is good. Fat is evil. Fat sustains. Fat kills. Fat nourishes. Fat destroys. Fat is a blessing. Fat burdens. Fat is attractive. Fat is ugly.

The fats in our diet are essential to sustain life. They nourish our nerve cells and are a key to having a healthy brain. Our bodies can synthesise most of our fats but we need linoleic and linoleinic acids and we can only get these through the food we eat. Without them, there is a breakdown of nerve cells and connective tissue and a malfunction of the brain. It is even suggested that, without adequate amounts of fat in our diets, dementia could be accelerated. The well-honed athlete at peak can look drawn and even emaciated as can the endurance runner or even the soccer player. Skinny catwalk models can look good in the right clothes and with the appropriate cosmetics but this physique is questionable when laid bare. In real life no one will argue with the look of the bonny, bouncing baby's body fat: we find ourselves oohing and gooing and admiring the chubby cheeks of our offspring.

Studies of the Yupik Eskimos in Alaska, who on average consume twenty times more omega 3 fats than people in other states of America suggest that a high intake of these fats helps to prevent obesity, heart disease and diabetes. This study was led by the Fred Hutchinson Cancer Research for Alaska Native Health Research at the University of Alaska, Fairbanks. This study also revealed that Type 2 diabetes was much lower than in the rest of America. Traditional lifestyle, refined foods and particular sugars are real killers. Fat is not the villain of our times but the saviour.

Street food, such as milk, butter, cheese and eggs, contrary to what we have been told in the past is actually good for us. All the studies of the people in this book and indeed across the world support this principle. Fat in moderation is good not evil. Porridge in the morning, a sandwich at lunch and meat and two vegetables in the evening, just like the diet of the ladies in our Fitness League, seem to be spot on. In fact, if we listen to Dr Aseem Malhotra, Honorary Consultant Cardiologist, he says that fat is our saviour and even lowers the level of cholesterol in our blood by as much as three times. Speaking at Croydon University, Malhotra even slammed the use of statins and claimed a diet high in saturated fat could protect rather than kill.

A Journal of American Medical Association study recently revealed that a low fat diet showed the greatest drop on energy expenditure and increased insulin resilience which is a precursor to diabetes. Dr Malhotra goes on to say that obesity in the States has rocketed despite the drop in calorie consumption falling from 40 percent to 30 percent, the reason being fats were replaced by sugar.

Professor Tim Noakes of the University of Cape Town has been saying for years that fats such as eggs and bacon are not the evil. It has taken forty years for America to realise that cholesterol in the blood is essential. The past studies on fatty diets and the subsequent evidence are one of the worst calamities in medical research.

This is backed up by the National Obesity Forum, chaired by Professor David Haslam, who said that the assumption has been made that increased saturated fat is the reason why we have the epidemic on obesity. Modern evidence is showing that it is not animal fat but refined food and particular sugar that is the main culprit, further supporting the claim about the worst medical error in our time.

OBESITY

Obese people can carry as much as a hundred billion fat cells in their body mass. A fat cell reaches it maximum capacity after puberty: when it reaches it maximum size the body will only produce more cells. Fat cells can be reduced in size through exercise and diet. Everyone carries fat. We have two kinds of fat: the white stuff that always seems to be around the waist and hips and the brown fat that allegedly is used to keep up warm in cold weather. We start to lose our brown fat when we become older and this is perhaps why we gather fat around the waist and hips in later life.

Genetics do play a part in how we accumulate fat but there is convincing evidence that exercise can play a part in controlling our body fat percentage. Research at Lund University Diabetes Centre in Sweden found that exercise switches on certain genes that have to do with fat storage.

World Cruiserweight Boxing Champion Archie Moore would often balloon between bouts. His answer to that when getting back in shape was to go on a diet of steak, chew it, and then spit it out before swallowing. He never failed to make the weight.

Elvis Presley believed in the Sleeping Beauty Diet. This meant being sedated for days; it worked because he never ate when sleeping. Losing weight does affect the brain. It was found that brain activity increases with weight loss. Obesity has been linked to several types of cancer. Being overweight causes cell changes in the body and losing weight will help in reducing arthritis.

Visceral fat (that's the fat around the intestines) can be reduced with dark chocolate but then again dark chocolate eaten in excess puts on weight. Lack of sleep makes it harder to lose weight and a daily can of soda increases the risk of obesity by 41%. Female breasts are almost entirely made up of fat and the eyelids are the only place that that we don't carry fat. There is also something called the 'Tapeworm Diet'. This means swallowing tapeworms to help lose weight. There is no limit to what people do to lose weight, all in the pursuit of looking better.

Shopping while hungry makes people buy more food. The psychological cause of this is our desire to survive. Science and common sense don't always see eye to eye. The answers in reality are very simple: eat less and move more but we are gifted with a brain and for that reason extend our thoughts and create quandaries. This is perhaps why dieting does not work and a change in attitude does.

All of this revolves around the principle that there is always a short cut or a quick fix but if we value our health, our life and a relatively stable existence then common sense, not science, should always triumph.

DEMENTIA

The saying that science never solves a problem without creating ten more is exemplified by the latest study on obesity, fat and dementia led by Dr Nawab Qizilbash, head of the clinical research organisation Oxon Epidemiology.

Qizilbash and his team combed through data on nearly two millions people in the United Kingdom Clinical Practice Research Datalink: The Medical Daily Report. Overall the people with a lower BMI than 20 faced a 34 percent higher risk of dementia than the ones who were overweight. What is not commented on in the report are the other characteristics and lifestyle habits of both underweight and overweight people. There seem to be some flaws in the study even though the results were conclusive.

The bottom line is that the risk of dementia is apparent with under- and overweight people. When studying the people in this book I saw little of the extremes: most were quite balanced, all were ageing, all were alert, even the ninety year olds, and all of them had a ritual of exercise in their daily or weekly lifestyle. Obesity is different from just being overweight. Being fat needs to start somewhere. Is it a dress size? Two inches on the trouser size? What about the degree of exercise or even the kind of exercise? Qizilbash's study does not really address these issues. For years we didn't acknowledge the difference between the different kinds of fat: now we know some of the differences.

'Being There' is a film made in 1979 starring Peter Sellers and Shirley MacLaine, adapted from the book of the same name, written by Jerzy Kosinski. It tells the story of a gardener who lives with his employers in an up market town house in Washington DC.

The main character is played by Sellers, a simple minded man who only knows gardening and what he sees on television. Chance (Sellers) is suddenly evicted onto the streets of the city with the death of his benefactors, the owners of the house. Dressed in a suit given to him by his wealthy master, Chance finds himself strolling the streets of the city. Stopping to look in a shop window he sees rows of televisions with one catching him on camera as he gazes at the goods inside. The surprise forces him to step back into the passing traffic where a chauffeur-driven limousine catches him and knocks him to the ground.

Full of apologies, the passengers jump out to comfort him. They help him to climb into the car and give him a drink to steady his nerves. The car owners, Ben Rand (Melvyn Douglas) and his wife Eve (Shirley MacLaine), drive him to their home to recover. When asked his name, Chance splutters 'Chance

Gardener.' The misinterpreted position of his name and his well-cut, expensive suit, combined with his old-fashioned manners create an image of a successful businessman.

The black comedy gathers pace when Chance starts to utter meaningless sentences about summer following spring and how saplings bend with the wind, planting seeds to grow our futures and other remarks about his garden. All this is mistakenly taken as a philosophy of a rich and successful business mogul. Rand and his young wife Eve believe that they have found a simple brand of true wisdom. Chance's comment that life is a state of mind sends Rand scurrying to the President, a connection he holds through his business.

Soon Chance Gardener is adviser to the Government. This is further enhanced by his familiarity with the President when he takes his hand in a consoling manner and calls him by his first name. Only people with a certain standard could easily slot into the realm of national and indeed world leaders.

The story is not unlike the fable The Emperor's New Clothes, another state of mind analogy. Chance is elevated to national prominence, making TV appearances and his simple words of wisdom soon resonates with the jaded American public. The story becomes even more bizarre when Rand announces that he is dying of aplastic anaemia, a form of dementia. He encourages his young wife Eve to get closer to Chance, which she does. When she kisses him, he responds because of his obsession with television movies and copies his idols. But Chance has no interest on sex. Eve, not realising that he is watching television, thinks he is talking to her when he says 'I like watching'. A little stunned but willing to follow her husband's advice, she starts to gyrate and simulates the sexual acts to satisfy his voyeuristic pleasure, not seeing that her efforts are going unnoticed as he watches TV.

Chance is present at Rand's death, after which he talks to

Rand's physician Dr Allenby. The doctor realises that Chance is just a simple-minded gardener who knows nothing of politics or finance. Allenby lets it go and makes no attempt to reveal the true extent of Chance's limited mentality. Perhaps in his wisdom he already knows that leadership and politics are led by people with little common sense after all.

The final scenes of the film show Chance watching the President's speech. The dark humour of the film implies that our simple gardener will be ready to step into the shoes of the President. The ironic scene shows Chance walking through Rand's estate, strengthening a bent pine sapling and then walking across a small lake. He pauses in the inch deep water, dips his brolly to measure the depth and turns to walk in the shallow depth appearing to be walking on water. The President of the United States watching, comments 'Life is a state of mind',

If the film had been made today the story could easily have been shown through the eyes of a dementia sufferer. Who is to know how we can interpret the inner working of our minds. We follow leadership unreservedly. The rantings of Trump are hardly the qualities of a sensible man. His derogatory language not once demonstrates wisdom that benefits a world at peace. It is not surprising that we the followers are blind to simplicity.

All the research in the world will never find a conclusive answer. The fictitious physician Dr Allenby saw little to be worried about with being led by a simple mind. The work on fat and omega 3 shows that there is a link between certain fats and obesity. There are also conclusive studies linking obesity and early death but not involving fat containing omega 3. Dementia and obesity are not conclusive but how much do they influence the eventual outcomes? Too much fat of any kind will spiral our body weight: fat studies show that too little fat can also affect not just our physical state but our mental capacity too.

DEMENTIA

These days, I am witnessing at first hand friends and colleagues who are victims of this terrible disease. Recently I met with a lifelong pal who is now on the slippery slope. He is someone who followed the rules: activity, sensible eating, constantly alert to do the right thing, a man surrounded by a loving family and real friends.

I see him regularly and the last time we talked at great length, mostly about life but always about the past. On entering the living room, I am greeted with a room full of music, Oscar Peterson's 'One more for the road' filling the air with melody, rhythm and the sound of excellent piano. My friend is now forsaking television, his walks are slower and his movements unsteady. We shared our humour, our interpretations of life and our sixty-five years of history. We shared the laughter, the tears and our philosophies of life. There is so little difference in our lives. His weight, like mine had differed only by small amounts. He has lifted, run, walked, swam and enjoyed his time in the past and now wonders like us all, what next? Like me, all his predecessors have gone: the remains of his past are a time to value. I tell this story because of the story about the film 'Being There' because that is where we are now: our wisdom is from our past, our experiences and our friendships.

Dementia is a part of life. Fat is a part of life. Obesity is a part of life. I look at my studies, the Fitness League and Lynn Ward's words of wisdom; Derek Craynor and Sylvia Faucitt and the hundreds who just eat three small meals a day. Nothing clever, no secrets except that they live by a code that embraces the chapters of this book: purpose, habits, rituals, their minds in the right place and a habit of continuity, consistency and doing what they set out to do. It might be a bit of a drag but they will do it anyway. All of them beyond the fads of eat fat and grow slim, low carbs, high carbs, low protein, high protein, the five a day, what's that, the Mediterranean diet? Well I do eat salad with my sandwich. Carry a bottle of water? What for? Pass the milk. What's wrong with a nice cup of tea? Dementia is a problem but for me not an unsolvable one. We do however need to focus; we need to embrace this challenge with the same verve with which we address our exercise programmes or our activity lifestyles. We need to look at it, give it our energy and our concentrated attention and, as is often the case, we need to find the simple solutions that evolve from our childhood.

Pussy cat, pussy cat where have you been?
I've been to London to see the Queen.
Pussy cat, pussy cat what did you there......

We all know how the story goes, but do we all know what it means?

I like the story of the cat and the Queen because it keeps reminding me of the need to get to where we want to go. We are all now in the battle to find our mental capacity, to keep pace with what we have done with our physical capacity. Dementia is the equivalent of sacrophenia, a wastage of muscle discussed in the Activity chapter.

The work started in the eighties and nineties on prolonging our physical state. People in their seventies, eighties and nineties fought any resistance in order to prolong their active lifestyles. The new frontier is now the brain and the works of Norman Doidge, Edward Taub and so many others who are forging new pathways, investigating the cells, synapses and neurons that keep our brains functioning.

Dementia is the modern day plague that is now into epidemic proportions. In order to challenge this disease we have to develop new methods and to develop new pathways. There is no one in a better position to do this than fitness trainers and those who exercise daily. Each of the characters in this book is already playing a part, each is contributing individually, though not yet collectively. From that very first visit to the Fitness League I knew that there was something special. It just needs harnessing along with all the other people putting it together. The jigsaw puzzle will give me a picture, and the picture will be of a brain that keeps reinventing itself, just as we keep warding off the threat of sacrophenia.

All of the characters I have met in this study are matched by millions out there who can add their knowledge and expertise to win this war. Longevity must be our aim but ultimately it must include having a quality of life that carries us past the hundred mark.

One such example of age and activity is Emma Morano, an Italian woman from the town of Verbania in North Italy. Emma has just celebrated her hundred and seventeenth birthday. Surviving two world wars and living in three different centuries, Emma is fully competent and, like all of our case studies, eats frugally. Her diet, if that is what we should call it, is even more simple than the other people in this book. She eats no fruit or vegetables. For many years she had three eggs a day, two of them being raw. Now her diet consists of a plate of minced meat, two eggs and some biscuits. There is little sign of dementia, but she has lost all her teeth. Emma Morano is one of eight children. She worked in a factory until the age of sixty-five and lives on the shores of Lake Maggiore. Dementia is not her problem, just handling old age. When being interviewed by the press and the verifier from the Guinness Book of Records, she asked if her hair was OK, pride and acceptability still being part of her respectability.

Fat, obesity and dementia are all synonymous with our lifestyle. Emma Morano, Ed Whitlock, Sylvia Faucitt, Derek Craynor, like all the others have a consistency. Yes they may be tempted to look under the chair or lose sight of what it is to stay active into old age, but there is a code of conduct: not to stray too far off the beaten track. So there is a pattern, a picture of what it looks like in the future, something that engages their imagination: a vision of how they will look when they are as old as Emma.

Throughout this study and the writing of this book there has been an underlying message, someone or something prodding away telling me what the secrets are. I know that we have to change and to do that we have to overcome fear, find purpose and develop new patterns of behaviour. We must keep pushing, keep going, ask questions, look around and try to absorb. I keep going back to go forward and the message from Lynn Ward about history holds true: without warning, another piece falls into place and bingo! I've got it and now I know where it's going and this is what will get us there.

23 – PLAN

Studies on the Longevity Project showed that stress was not a factor in illness and premature death. What came out was that hard work and helping others was more important than diet and exercise. Other important factors were having good friends, meaningful and strong community involvement and social networking.

The study goes on to say that people who plan their life around a healthy lifestyle are in effect enriching their future. John Higson, Derek Craynor and many of those in our People chapter are prime examples of people making their own luck. The Longevity Project, conducted by Howard S Friedman from the University of California, found that attitude plays a huge part in not just our lifespan but our resistance to disease.

John Higson said 'I made my mind up at the age of 24 to live to be a hundred.' Sylvia Faucitt, who broke her neck, said 'I don't look for excuses to stop, but reasons to continue.' These two people are among the many in this book who are by design long-livers and who are active in the old age because of their attitude.

Another study, the National Preventative Strategy in the USA, is one of the most ambitious programmes in the world. The lifestyles of the people in this study are mirrored in the characters in this book. The National Preventative study and mine agree that communities and tribes are vital in warding off disease, in fostering a healthy outlook and a conscious effort to eat well, but no one is clear on how we can create our own community or tribe.

There is also strong evidence to show that our genetic inheritance is responsible for just 25% of our health, well-being and longevity which suggests that we have more control over our destiny than previously thought.

Another factor that came out of these studies was that exercise and hard work effected the hippocampus, that part of the brain that promotes good health. Wendy Suzuki, a Professor of Neuroscience and Psychology at New York University Centre for Neuroscience, spoke on the Ted Talks programme about Neuroplasticity which we know is the brain's ability to remould itself. Suzuki's principles include positive affirmations during exercise. These visual and vocal methods improve the brain's ability to both develop new cells and perform better. These studies, and the ones by Norman Doidge in his book 'The Brain That Changes Itself', are consistent with the people in this book and the information in the Longevity Project and the National Prevention Strategy.

The Women's League of Health and Beauty was formed in the 1930s, it was based on strict adherence to a discipline of a correct exercise routine, posture and military drills. Over recent years the military philosophy has changed but the mindset is still the same. This mindset, strict attention to technique and a repetitive message install a sense of trust: we believe in what we do, which was the philosophy that came out of my interviews.

All four of these studies have two common denominators and those are that we are subject to regularity, be it work or exercise and that we need to think about what we do. Our attitude to life dictates our future and to drift through life only makes us one of the herd. To plan is to think and to think puts us among the ones we call the tribe.

FINDING YOUR TRIBE

It was just 15 years of age when I joined my first gym. The gym was in an old cinema that had seen better days showing silent films. The days of Greta Garbo, Charlie Chaplin, Lillian Gish, Douglas Fairbanks and Rudolph Valentino were passing into history and the old King's Hall was welcoming the seeds of a new era of fitness.

The war had ended just five years before and it was here that I found my peace of mind, the security of a welcoming group and an extended family of like thinkers. I had, in simple terms, found my tribe. A young kid among men who were strength athletes of immense power, of great reputation with hearts and personalities that matched their status: Jumping Jim Halliday, a British and Commonwealth Champion, Syd Baker, a County and Northern County Champion, Abe Greenhalgh and Jack Lord, all champions who in my eyes matched the stars of the silent screen.

Now at 81 years of age and 67 years a member of the tribe, I can still feel the security, the satisfaction and the sense of being part of something bigger than us all. I was lucky to have found my tribe early and I would roam the plains of life with many thousands of other members but the ethos, beliefs and instincts would prevail for generation after generation.

Tribes come in all shapes and sizes. They are out there. They are welcoming, helpful and provide a variety to your life. They are all about us, if we care to look and make an effort to seek them out. They come packaged in all sizes and shapes and are called by different names. Some call themselves clubs: 'Connie' clubs, Labour clubs, health clubs, bowling clubs, cricket clubs and soccer clubs. Some call themselves groups: networking groups, business groups, social groups, walking groups and political groups. There are groups within groups, sometimes five, six or seven, sometimes thousands. There are Internet groups, Twitter groups, Facebook groups, but the best of all are the groups that laugh together, cry together, drink, eat and smile together and yes even pray together. Not all groups, not all tribes have these qualities.

Look for like-minded people. When we started in business and tried to make a livelihood out of running a gym, it was a natural transition from having a hobby to making it a profession. My immediate thoughts when starting this huge change in our lives was to go back to basics and remember how I was welcomed into the old silent cinema called the King's Hall. It was here that we had an old dilapidated building; the only equipment was basic weights, dumbbells, barbells; no showers or changing rooms, no lockers. What it did have was heart and soul and an atmosphere that embraced all of us. This, I knew, was what was needed when starting the business in the world of fitness.

Our new club had all the luxuries: carpets, equipment that was modern and well-made. We had changing rooms, showers, lockers, a restaurant, a crèche for the children and a beauty salon. Plants decorated the reception area, the coffee bar and cafe. All would have stood for nothing if we had not put in the heart and soul: the welcome and the invitation to join our tribe.

It is now over forty years since the start of that club, and there is hardly a day goes by without me being reminded of how people felt about being part of our tribe. We can provide all the material comforts of life, but we can never beat how people care or feel about us and our involvement in the club. People, almost half a century on, remind me about what they felt about their club, not mine, about their involvement and their happy times. People don't care who you are, what you have, or why you're here. They only care how much you care and that is the most fundamental quality that makes up the tribe and separates it from the herd. So when choosing your tribe, it is not how much you can get but how much you can give.

Group dynamics play a huge part in the workings of our society, in business, sport and family life. How we integrate, socialise and support each other is fundamental to any group's success. Not all groups work. They fail in business and in sport and they fail in family. Finding that balance can be a huge challenge and is not always possible in one's working life or even in the family. The tribe that you need meets the needs of the individual and that individual is you.

When Wynne Barber, one of my case studies, left the army in 1945, she immediately thought of the Women's League of Health and Fitness.

'I wanted freedom of movement and music', she said.

She also wanted the freedom of expression. The disciplines of the war were replaced by the easier disciplines of the Women's League of Health and Fitness.

John Higson when being interviewed said 'I worked hard all my life.'

Higson's escape was his work.

When seeking your tribe, look for the compatibility of others, people you feel comfortable with, groups that fit your needs and have a similar interest, or just those who are good to chat with. The strength of your tribe is summed up in the strength of your needs and how comfortable you feel in the group.

In the current world of technology it is easier to form groups online. This can have the effect of disassociating ourselves from the realistic view of what tribe means. Texts, emails, Facebook and the using of other forms of communication eliminate the social skills that occur when face to face. Social interactions when face to face abound with mannerisms: eye contact, body language, rapport, a smile, a frown, a shift in position, a nod of the head, a shake of the head, a glance away and many other nuances that make up our verbal and non-verbal language. Everybody tells a story when face to face, even when there is no vocal conversation.

In today's world of communication, technology is of great importance but not in terms of emotional connection: so much is lost in interpretation when expression is left solely to the written word. Yes, we can talk but to forge friendships, emotional connection and trust then we need to be face to face. When people of Great Britain voted to leave the European Union it was because the emotional connection had been severed. The head of the tribe had become disassociated from just one part of the body and that part of the body simply lost trust in the tribe leader's ability to lead.

Great Britain's huge success in the 2016 Olympic Games shocked and sent shivers through the athletic and political world. Few recognised why and how it had happened. This small island with a population of just 50 million had produced so much success and yet countries like China, India, Russia and America had failed to compare.

Many would appreciate the thought, the planning and the attention to detail; many would say it was the funding, the Lottery money; some would lay suspicion on the darker side of performance. Fewer people would appreciate the instincts of the tribe and the growing psychology that had started ten years before at the home of British Cycling, the Velodrome in Manchester. Dave Brailsford and his counterparts formed the nucleus of this new intelligence and the start of a mindset that would spread, eventually, to every part of the British contingent. Not many then would appreciate the attention to detail, the philosophy of marginal gains and no stone unturned.

A decade later it was the diminutive former Olympian, Victoria Pendleton, who said on TV at the close of the 2016 Olympics:

'We now have systems: everyone who joins us knows exactly what to do.'

This is the result of ten years: ten years of development, ten years of margins, food, energy expedition, supplementary training. Preparation, preparation, preparation: the tribe within the tribe developing the instincts and intelligently steering the remainder to a better, more productive and safer existence.

The difference between tribes and herds is in one word: intelligence. The tribe needs leadership; the herds just drift. The tribes build trust; the herds stampede. The Tribe develops, cultures systems and a mindset; the herd just exists.

When planning your future, remember to include the groups of people who have similarities to you. Search for your tribe and plan.

24 – CHALLENGE

FATNESS KILLS

Statistics demonstrate over and over again that being over-weight leads to diabetes. Diabetes leads to heart disease and heart disease leads to death.

That rather over-simplistic statement leads to complicated questions but the truth is that it is right. Fat in excess kills. It also leads to a deterioration of our mental capacity and that in turn leads to dementia. Nothing is that simple nor is finding a solution but the fact is that fat or no fat, we are entering a time of real crisis. Finding an answer to dementia is probably the greatest challenge of modern times. We are all living longer and we are all subject to this modern plague and right now no one has an answer for our children and our children's children as to what we should do about it.

This is not for us. At eighty-two years of age, my concern is not for now but for our future generations. That said, the need to commit is not just a problem for governments, but a problem for each of us to join in and fight the fight, right here in our own back yard.

In each of these chapters there are ingredients to keep our bodies and our minds in shape. This was never a book to address longevity: it is to provide an answer to the issue of keeping people fit, healthy and vigorous to the end of our life. I do believe that the people in this book and the study over the last year, and my previous sixty years in fitness, proves that people can remain active. What I didn't expect was that not only did these people prove that we can stay physically active but also that we can enjoy sanity till the end.

Each chapter provides us with the start to a solution: we first have to overcome the fear of doing something to resolve the problem. We as individuals need to look at this from a point of unconscious incompetence. We do not know what this is but the challenge to change is within us all, as is the fear of change. What we do know, however, is that the brain needs to be challenged. We do know that if a muscle in the arm is to grow, it needs to be worked on and to work we challenge it. I have spent a lifetime challenging people to escape from their comfort zones. The same principle in challenging our physical capacity applies to challenging our mental capacity. Only by overcoming our fear of commitment will we find an answer to any of our problems, let alone to dementia.

I had almost finished this book before I realised how close we are to solving the onset of dementia. The first hint of this was when I told the story of the racing driver, Tom Bradshaw and I realised that the programme for Tom came so close to working the brain just as much as the body. My task with Tom was to develop hand to eye contact and develop eye to feet contact. The programme is as relevant to challenging the brain for motor racing as it is to developing new brain cells to stave off dementia. The programme, with some adjustment, will create cells, neurons, synapses and pathways.

Edward Taub, Norman Doidge and Michael Merzenich have made great progress in dealing with stroke and brain trauma patients. What is now evident is that the physical side of these studies should be combined with the social involvement of people who are telling us that both the body and the brain can work progressively to achieve similar goals.

There is very little of this book that relied on any form of linked study. In fact it was the opposite. Almost everyone, every character, came out of a peripheral view. I didn't know what I was looking for and in not knowing that, I accepted unconditionally what I was being told. It has been my job over the past twelve months to piece this information together and try to make sense of it all and then one day I had that blinding flash of the obvious gave me a eureka moment.

THE NON-SEQUENTIAL BRAIN

Sophia Rose Thorpe was just five months old. Both Sophia and myself were having a conversation about neuroplasticity. I knew she understood every word I said because those beautiful little eyes were all over the place, her arms and her legs were constantly moving, she was giggling and smiling and the large television screen to the side was also catching her attention. Sophia's little brain was randomly absorbing all this and she was also absorbing her great-grandfather's words without knowing what the words meant. This is at the time of her life when the brain is at its height in absorbing and storing information. At some time in the future, her growing brain will sort out the wheat from the chaff and my gibberish will go in the waste bin; or will it?

The brain is not challenged by logic nor will it grow linearly. The brain grows new cells by being surprised by random pieces of information. The human race evolved over time without plans, strategies or logical processing. It grew because it was forced to grow to survive the fight, to flee or to freeze. It was born and developed out of non-sequential activity. To grow these cells we need to surprise them.

Habits and rituals fulfil a purpose in our lives. They provide the essential structure and reliability that we need. It was said in the film 'Snowden' that people don't want freedom, they want security and that is why communism thrives and dictatorships work. The human race showed their individuality when they voted for Brexit and for Trump, and proved that freedom of thought will change things. This is where and why a child's brain will ask for nothing more than constant change and random growth.

It would be another week before I realised how much that talk with our great-granddaughter meant. The words of Derek Craynor and Mary McDaid popped into my head. 'To rest is to rust,' he said. Not resting and constant activity develop new cells and Mary's philosophy confirmed it. The never-ending change of classes and choreography keeps the brain active and on edge and to have that in the environment of friendship and a social structure of good habits and the ritualistic approach fulfils most of the essentials. The brain and the body are closely related. Thinking and moving stimulate the body's need for circulation, blood flows to every area including the brain and to make the brain work separately when at the same time moving the body creates maximum benefit.

This is far more effective than doing crossword puzzles, Sudoku or computer games. Each of them will help but activity is far more beneficial with movement, company, friendship, conversation and the security of tribe. If we could dovetail crosswords with physical exercise then you would probably have a perfect answer and that maybe the future but right now The Fitness League, Derek Craynor and my great-granddaughter Sophia Rose are all waging war on the monster dementia. Between us all, we will slay the beast.

GOASTING

Some years ago, Brenda and I, along with Jonah and Madeleine Barrington were supposed to be on holiday, but Jonah and Madeleine wanted to sample the regime of being a marathon runner. We would run each morning and then later we would run in the early evening. Marathon runners will cover over a hundred miles a week with this method, so both of them accompanied me on my own particular ritual.

Jonah was recovering from an elbow operation, so his squash was forbidden. Thus the running provided a good alternative to his limited ritual. But Jonah had an insatiable appetite for training: like me he never played at anything. To suggest that he should take a rest was unthinkable. Why would I not do this when I am capable? The fact that he could not play the game of squash was no excuse not to practise the game of squash; so Jonah came up with one of the most torturous substitutes ever devised. He came up with something he called 'goasting'.

Goasting would normally be done on a regular squash court and because there were no courts at our hotel, we made do with drawing the floor of a court in the grounds of the hotel's gardens. Goasting is like the equivalent of shadow boxing that fighters do with an imaginary opponent. We mapped the court out on the grass complete with serving boxes and the appropriate dimensions of a full grown court. The idea was to force the player to simulate the movement in six different parts of the court. The two front corners, the back two corners and the two serving boxes on each side of the T. The coach (me) would have a stop watch and I would shout out at random, a number that related to the six points of the court. The player (Jonah) would then hurry and scurry across the court at high speed while I counted how many stations he covered in a ninety second period. HIIT on a squash court. The year was 1984.

The exercise of goasting was to develop speed of movement, agility and bodily stamina. What we didn't know then was that it was also developing the new brain cells in a part of the brain called the frontotemporal. Goasting is not an exercise for the ageing population: it is an incredibly challenging exercise to do, requiring speed, fast movement and agility of both body and mind. I would not recommend it to anyone over the age of fifty nor perhaps even younger. Knees, lower back, ankles and quads are all near to trauma but for the brain? It's unbeatable. To make this principle work for our ageing warriors we need to have a console on, say, a bike that demands the simulation on a touch pad.

Speed of thought is not a necessity when sharpening and developing our brain cells. Constant change is probably needed, purpose and importantly mixing with people. We should never underestimate family, friends, and, as Olga Brown, one of our case studies, said 'Love'. Olga, who plays netball, swims and does pilates, is at eighty years of age a prime example of what this book is about. None of the people in the book lack attitude or have special diets. They are, however, positive in their approach and by some strange phenomenon agree with each other. This was evident when I first visited the Fitness League at St Osmund's: I sensed a form of telepathy, an uncanny communication that everyone inside or outside the Fitness League seem to have.

Jonah Barrington's goasting was not intended to sharpen his brain but was conducted to sharpen his stamina. Jonah found out early in his career that he lacked that edge when he needed that speed. Once he knew this, he trained to outlast his opponents and develop the percentage game. Jonah, like all of us, has some natural weakness and for the six times World Champion it was a lack of pace. On discovering this, he trained to wear his opponents down by constantly pressing them just as how teams are pressed in soccer. We cannot change our DNA, no more than we can change the dead brain cells of our ageing brains, but we can create new ones and this is achieved by challenging them.

Governments across the world have known for over fifty years that we would have this enormous problem with dementia because of the baby boom between 1946 and the 60s. In those years the expected life span was three score years and ten. That would predictably rise: the estimated life span now stands at three score years and seventeen or even higher. In other words seventy-eight, even eighty or eight-two years of age. The United Nations estimated that there are 316,600 people living to be a hundred worldwide, and one in every three babies will live to be over that age. The United States, according to the 2010 census, has more than 53,000 people living to be over a hundred. Japan has the second largest with over 51,000 living to that age. Our Queen Mother lived to be a hundred and two years of age and our own Queen Elizabeth has just celebrated her ninetieth birthday, with Prince Philip now at ninety-five. Longevity is real and so is dementia and if we are to address this catastrophic problem then we and our governments have to address it now.

INNOVATION

Significant and positive change is not just needed to find a solution to the inevitable problem, it is essential. Finding an answer cannot be left to science alone: industry leaders, educational institutions and particularly legislation from governments should free the restriction of protocol. Dementia is not just a disease, it is war. In just fifty years time, we will be faced with zombie-like nations with a third of our ageing people unable to understand anything. Long term studies will not stop the blitz of short term invasion of our senses. The challenge for a saner future is the responsibility of all.

On the third of September 1939 Neville Chamberlain, the Prime Minister of Britain, announced at 11.15 am that

England and France had declared war on Germany. Over sixty million people would die over the following six years and many more would be maimed and die as a result of the conflict. Premature death would follow from gas poisoning, shell shock, gangrene, post war trauma, depression and suicide. Without the state of emergency declared in 1939 the total number of casualties would have been even more catastrophic. Now, with the creeping rigor mortis of dementia and its associated issues, we have a new war that is even greater. The time is not now. NOW is the time to act and so is the challenge.

Innovation is usually a term associated with business and right now the business of fitness is poised to address this global problem. Just as it is poised, it is also immature. The corporations are money-driven as expected. Maturity always comes at a price: innovative programmes designed to challenge our brains are not even in the minority. They are nonexistent. Personal trainers are motivated by fashionable trends; clubs push short term satisfaction and neglect education. The average customer knows little about fitness, progressive resistance, V^o2 max, body fat percentage, health-related and fitness-related injuries. Diabetes is for the newspaper articles, fitness magazines or the latest flier announcing a new class. We are like sheep in that we follow fads and trends, fashionable and commercial innovations, not health or the latest research. If we did we would be asking our watches, our phones, laptops and apps, what we do to be alert at sixty or seventy years of age, but because this four billion pound industry panders to the young, they skirt around the real issues of health. They do meaningless MOTs, blood pressure, obesity, pulse rate and sometimes height, and guesstimate the results. There is little real expertise because real expertise is an unknown quantity: science and the commercial world of fitness are a million miles apart for the simple reason that governments, medicine and science all work independently. They stand and watch a sinking ship drowning in apathy. The oxymoron approach to health is not studying health it is studying sickness.

There is no recognised strategy for preventing dementia and its associated Alzheimer's Disease, yet there are an approximate 46.8 million people worldwide who suffer from the disease. Alzheimer's Disease International (ADI) along with Bupa are often called the voice of Alzheimer's. ADI estimate that by the year 2050 there will be over a hundred and thirty million people with dementia in America alone. The cost to the nation now is eight hundred and eighteen billion dollars, and is expected to be a trillion dollar figure by 2018. This is a bigger threat than ISIS, bigger than the wars in the East, bigger than all the collective terrorist groups in the world put together. All the reports across the world give no indication that a cure is either imminent or in the future. Not one of the organisations in the hundred and four countries across the world has even one suggestion that will help to prevent dementia or Alzheimer's. The world doesn't have a cure nor does it have a preventative policy.

COLLABORATION

If we are to even touch the surface of the biggest threat since World War II, then science and physical fitness should get together. Innovation will drive business and even science only because the end product is profit but the bottom line here is costing everyone a loss on all of our balance sheets, not just on the financial spread sheets but on the cost of care, medicine, sickness and health. We need to bring our international sports coaches and put them on the same tables as Edwards Taub, Norman Doidge and the other top neuroscientists in the world. We have to change our mentality first before we change the world. We need to go back to basics and listen to what the cat saw and realise that if we go to London to see the Queen, then we can't look at the next meal. The simple solution is staring us in the face; the complicated one's looking in the wrong direction. The grey cells need exercise.

KNOWING WHAT WE DON'T KNOW

It was Albert Einstein who said that there is nothing new, it has all been done before, we just need to reach out and find it. I have spent over sixty years studying health and fitness, so when starting this book and meeting the people, I had to start with no preconceived ideas about what I was looking for. I thought in the beginning that I knew and I found out that I didn't.

I them remembered the battle at Marks and Spencer for Stuart Rose was a bitter and tumultuous war with his once rival Philip Green, which he subsequently won. Soon after the dust had settled Philip Green was asked about his defeat and how Stuart Rose would cope.

'He will do the job' said Green, 'because he knows what he doesn't know.'

The true secret of leadership is knowing what your failing are and finding compensation to manage them. Philip Green knew Rose would surround himself with good lieutenants just as every good general would do in war. The challenge for Rose would be the same challenge for Green, and the challenge for us is to cure dementia or at least stave off the onset.

It is little use sticking ardently to something that doesn't achieve results. We know that the Fitness League gets results because it has history. Lynn Ward told me that and I couldn't see it. 'History,' she said, 'it's been around since 1932: of course it's got history.' Here I am now and Ann Hunt leads the class and thirty people remember every single move when they should have lost their minds and haven't. That class is being repeated all over the world, in Canada, Holland, New Zealand, Australia, and like the three hundred other classes in this country, they will have a 90 year old exercising to the sound of Heather Small or Sam Smith.

Wow! That statistic needs looking at.

I am now in my seventh decade of study and I can't get over Derek Craynor, his jam butties, cauliflower ear and his unbelievable vigour and enthusiasm. Like John Higson, Sylvia Faucitt and Wynne Barber's merlot or Ed Whitlock's tea and toast and sub four hour marathons. I can not help but listen to Mary from County Wicklow and how she gets her class to work their brains; and eighty-four year old Tony Ford who thought he's had it at seventy-eight. 'The answers are there,' said Einstein, 'now we just need to find them'; and I have. Our challenge is to find more of these people; people in the past such as Billy Leach, Joe Heathcote, Bert Loveday and our friends in Oregon, Bill and Judy Pearl. They too, like the people here, are staving off dementia; they are still in the gym. They too, like the others, have fought their way through the years, sometimes pushing to their limits, sometimes nurturing their aches and pains, overcoming the challenges of live, meeting them and then not expecting favours, but ready for the next whatever it may be. God, I am so lucky to be in their presence.

We here in Bolton, live approximately six thousand miles from our friends in Talent, Oregon. We have known the Pearls now for nearly fifty years. Bill is now eighty-six years of age and he and his wife Judy walk across from their ranch home and enter their gym, which they call the Barn.

'We do that four times a week,' Bill tells me. 'We train for about one and a half hours per session and somehow we work around the wear and tear.'

Bill's whole career was about bodybuilding: four times Mr Universe, Mr US and Mr America, the World's Best Built Man, the titles go on.

Their barn attracts a different clientele now than it did on my last visit. The demographics have changed. When I was last there they were all into training competitions, big chests and big arms; now the average age is in the seventies; they have replacement knees and hips, and train to keep their equilibrium , and with balance being one of the things we lose in our seventies, we have learned to adapt. Training today at eighty-six, means balancing the energy better, the effort better and a better way of controlling our physical assets.

'We can't do it like we used to, Kenny,' he said.

Pearl's commitment over the years with heavy and punishing workouts has been a constant challenge on his frame, his muscle and the joints of his skeletal frame. Still in great shape, active in this lifestyle, Pearl is an example how we can balance our life through good nutrition, positive attitude and being active into old age. The challenge for Pearl was doing all of that and still achieving the heights he did.

PREVENTION

Intercept means to divert, avoid, change course, re-route or avert. This book started with a clear objective: I knew exactly what I wanted to achieve, which was for people to enjoy and fill the latter days of their lives with energy, vigour and a feeling of fulfilment. I was soon to find out that these people I was interviewing were telling me far more than I had bargained for. My preconceived idea was being forced to change. The problem was I wasn't seeing it: I didn't know what I didn't know. Well that was until the penny dropped. My mind, like the cat's, was elsewhere until I suddenly realised that it wasn't what they said but what they were not saying.

I have been asking questions for most of my adult life; questions that need specific answers. The answers to certain questions would tell me what my clients wanted from us, whether it was to slim or to build up or other ambitions related to fitness. People rarely open up to sensitive questions: losing weight can mean looking good on the beach or being toned with shapely shoulders. The ladies will see themselves gracefully making their entrance onto the poolside with admiring eyes from both men and women. The men see abs, biceps and a V-shaped back. People came into our clubs to enhance their physical assets not to buy shoes, clothes or fish and chips: they came to either look good or feel good. It was my job and our staff's jobs to get into the mind of our prospective customer: we were successful at providing an answer for over thirty years and made many friends along the way, many of which are still around to remind us.

Those years of practice helped me to intercept the answers to my questions about life style and why they were doing what they were doing at seventy, eighty and even ninety years of age. This time, however, I missed the real secret of what kept them physically and mentally fit, healthy and mentally alert with hardly a hint of dementia. There is no doubt in my mind that almost all of these people in our case studies are following the basic rules that are outlined in most of the studies on neuroplasticity. It was obvious to me that what our neuroscientists are saying is that exercise in a congenial environment that challenges the brain to think does in fact develop new neurological pathways, even when walking. Walking alone, however, is not enough: we need to engage the mind at the same time. One of the world's most respected neuroscientists, Professor Michael Merzenich, recommends looking at your environment, looking at things in a new light, seeing the flowers, seeing your environment as though you have never seen it before. Walking will provide the physical involvement but it is your mental awareness that helps to develop the brain cells. Installing a positive mental attitude for just twenty minutes in a one hour exercise programme will over time get results.

HOW TO CHALLENGE THE BRAIN

All of the exercises in our Activity chapter are capable of developing brain cells. To make them work we isolate the thinking from the doing. Wearing headphones is good if you want to pass the time, but if you want to improve your brain then dump the music. Watches are ok if you need to know the time, but if your want to develop new brain pathways, then dump the watch. The only sure way of developing new brain cells is to work with the brain when active.

Prof Michael Merzenich at the University of California, San Francisco, will say that we have to be there in the moment with the mind and body in sync. In other words, we need to be in the zone when building new cells that just may help us to prevent us from suffering dementia.

Weight training, bowls, running or rambling and all the physical activities listed in our Activity chapter will set us on the road to a better life. Merzenich, speaking on TED Talks, says it's all about change, and like our great-granddaughter, it all comes down to the example of learning by constantly using change as a tool to keep developing our brain cells. Curiosity, seeing things in a refreshing way, trying new things, new classes, new choreography, new routines, and even new ways to do old exercises. Try a zottman curl, a two hands snatch, install fresh thinking into a spin class, challenge the brain, surprise the brain, think fresh, think new, think differently.

WALKING FOOTBALL

The Fitness League started in 1932. Mary Baggott Stack created history that may just go on and on and like our ageing population the league will live to be more than a hundred years of age. What I have learned from them is that body and brain and exercise are so closely related that they become inseparable. This only happens, however, when we make it happen. Perhaps Mary Baggott Stack knew this when she looked at the concept in Germany in the late twenties. Certainly no one nor any of the literature have drawn reference to this but there is a distinct link.

Edward Taub, Norman Doidge and the Neuroscientists across the world are pioneering the development of new brain cells. The Fitness League are, and have been, at the stage of unconscious competence. They are doing it but they don't know they are doing it. Ann Hunt here in Bolton and her compatriots across the world need to think about how they can improve what they are already doing. This is a simple skill of making their classes perform more complicated moves and they need to explain this to their fun-loving members. They still need the fun. 'They can do this forever,' said Sally Floyd. How right she was to teach them to think more and develop the brain more for Mary McDaid. We are all just starting on this journey and that includes soccer.

Walking Football has so many things in common with the Fitness League that it seems almost untrue. But it is. The potential of this phenomenon is limitless. Both of these concepts are designed to work. Both brain and body move us and shake us, test us and at the same time, allow us to have fun.

There are lots of rules to walking football, lots of things to remember. Having learned the rules, the player progresses to the stage of unconscious competence. It is at this stage or even before that, that the professional coach uses his or her ability to install new memory skills to keep the brain and the cells working. Walking football contains all the ingredients, exercise, congeniality, tribe, purpose and FUN. A place to be, to enjoy and to be active in both body and mind.

MIND CHANGING

I started this book knowing what had to be said. My intentions were to write the narrative around four main areas: diet, exercise, mind and tribe. Within the first thirty days of interviews and research, I was already seeing it differently. By the time I had put pen to paper the story line, or the journey, was off on a tangent. People were telling me to change course; food was not the prerogative, nor was the exercise. Both, although not irrelevant, were of less importance than company, congeniality and comfortable surroundings. Tribe was starting to take preference.

By the end of the first ninety days, I had met up with the first hundred people and what was coming back from them was more about mentality than about activity. Derek Craynor put me in my place when I watched him work out. My mind was asking questions, challenging me to think. Derek was defying all the rules: technique, order of exercise, a mismatch of sequence. Sugar Puffs for breakfast, jam sandwich before training. I am supposed to be the expert here!

Then Lynn Ward's history? Then thirty odd women and not one mentioning the Mediterranean diet, or five a day. Cereal for breakfast, sandwich for lunch. Doris Hughes, at ninety years old, belting it out to Heather Small. Laughter.

Friendship. Then another turning point in the book with Mary McDaid's left and right brain and the realisation that there is more in the mind than in the body. Edward Taub, Bill Pearl, Norman Doidge, Sally Floyd; they can do this for ever. Then a defining moment with Sam Smith and Ann Hunt's choreographed sequence that captured the essence of a concentrated mind and a complicated move. This time not the mind, but the brain, had to work memorising recently formulated drills, movement, timing, rhythm, physical and mental demand simultaneously.

What are they all saying? How can they tell me if they don't know? A piece here, a line, sentence:

'If you rest you rust.' Change, constant change.

'It comes from within,' said Billy.

'It's been working for eighty-five years,' said Lynne.

'Challenge the brain,' said Mary.

'Neuroplasticity works,' said Norman Doidge.

Ninety billion neurons, the hippocampus, new pathways, synapses, new cells and the brain demanding to be worked.

Sophia Rose Thorpe, at five months old, absorbing every movement, soaking up the environment; sound, touch, sight, smell, tasting everything and everything.

A challenge, arms, legs, eyes, body, muscle, tendon, heart and lungs; the six senses working hard to tell me what next.

The secrets are there in each of the characters; from the scientists to our ladies and men who know the answers and don't know that they know.

Perhaps we collectively can join the dots through the chapters of this book.

'The answers are there,' said Albert Einstein, 'we just have to reach out and find them.'

What can we learn from these wonderful people? Each of them is telling us something that leads to changing the way that our minds, our brains and even our DNA work. Only a few of the people in this book are super athletes: Bill Pearl, Ed Whitlock, and Ulrich Inderbinen. The other thousands who I researched are just ordinary people who have somehow found the elixir of youth.

Each of them is demonstrating this by example but when I ask them what it is that works, they modestly shrug or relate a saying or mantra:

'If you rest you rust,' said Derek Craynor.

'History,' said Lynne Ward.

Billy Leach: 'Health comes from within.'

'The left and right side of the brain,' said Mary McDaid.

And Ed Whitlock's 'I find training a drag'.

The clues to a vigorously long life are in each of our friends, colleagues and characters in this book. All that we have to do is join up the dots and the dots are right here in the chapters of this book. Think collectively, think individually, ask yourself what does each chapter say and how is it explained through the characters of this book. Only then will you have your answer to how you can find the secrets to eternal youth and yes, live forever.

25 – FUTURE

The late nineteen seventies saw a vast number of major changes that at the time were quite unrelated. Dr Kenneth H Cooper, a retired Air Force colonel, invented the term 'aerobics'. This word would relate to something called 'exercise to music'. While this was happening, Bob Geldof, of the rock and punk band called The Boomtown Rats, would change the world with one of the biggest charity events ever. The word 'leisure' would describe something that we did when we had nothing else to do which became a global market that is now worth over five hundred billion dollars. The late seventies and early eighties would transform our world: whole industries that had survived and flourished would give away to a leisurely fashionable industry that would affect our lives in a thousand different ways and fitness would find its identity.

I always felt that the influence of dance spawned the emergence of aerobics. Olivia Newton John and John Travolta's 'Saturday Night Fever' and 'Grease' started the dance craze and this spilled over into exercise to music which in turn started the fashion craze of leotards, head bands, wrist bands and leg warmers, then exploded into entertainment. Jane Fonda starred in a film called 'Workout' that sold as an exercise class and a catchphrase 'Go for the burn'. All these developments helped our business at the health club in Bolton. The boom in aerobics would help to make our business sexy. It was cool to do exercise, our profile would escalate and with that a desire to provide a reputable service. The reputation would spark a conscience to do more for our customers and that would lead to a greater responsibility to achieve results and it would be the results that would define our business.

The start of the running boom began in the mid seventies. By 1980, the London Marathon was attracting thousands. My first marathon, the Preston to Morecambe in 1975, comprised just thirty-seven runners. By 1980, we had twenty runners training at our bodybuilding club called Bolton Health Studio, they all had times of under three hours, and every one of them was over forty years of age. These people, our members, were not athletes: they worked in industry, they were shop keepers, business men, bus drivers and butchers, bakers and candlestick makers. Well not quite but you get my meaning.

RESULTS

Results mattered then and results matter now. The phenomenon of non-runners achieving runners' times fascinated me. We had had plenty of success that we took for granted: we didn't really ask why. Our business would grow and with that our desire to find out why. It was about this time that I began to explore just how much the mind played in these ordinary people achieving extraordinary results. There were two things specifically that changed the way I thought: one was the book by Robert Ornstein and David Sobel 'The Healing Brain' and the other was discovering Neuro Linguistic Programming (NLP). The former was a prelude to neuroplasticity before anyone gave it a name. The later is all about communication through our senses. Both these things in the eighties were still in their infancy but both are now accepted methods of science. Both could be a prelude to what is next.

There is a saying in business that we cannot manage what we cannot measure: sport is a great example of this. Times, distance, tables and results; the first over the line, through the tape, the top of the table; and the hundreds of different tools to measure performance. But as yet, nothing measures the mind. This fascination with how the mind works would challenge me to test myself both physically and mentally.

On my fortieth birthday I ran forty miles, then I immediately followed this by lifting forty thousand pounds in a period of forty minutes. On completing that I went onto the squash court and played four different people, one after the other, each to the best of five games. The forth and final challenge of my fortieth birthday was to do four hundred sit-ups. This was at a time when all the medical recommendations were to slow down our lives at forty. This was also at a time when squash was a game to avoid for fear of a heart attack, when weightlifting was considered the same and when running forty miles was just for bizarre and weird people who ran themselves into the ground and invited collapse. The four hundred continuous sit-ups were really just there to add insult to injury. Here's the twist. I did it all again on my fiftieth. Ten years later, ten years older, and all four disciplines in units of five or fifty. Fifty miles, fifty thousand pounds in weights in fifty minutes, five people at squash, and five hundred sit-ups. No sign of collapse, no extreme fatigue, no special food drinks and no mental trauma.

SPECIFICS, REPETITION, EXPECTATION

Training for any event requires levels of concentration. We don't train someone to run marathons by prescribing sprints, nor do we train a boxer by putting her or him onto a wresting mat. Training to be a footballer demands football training. We don't prepare our children by not being specific: exams are not passed for economics by teaching history. We define our subject and repeatedly focus on the topic, speciality or subject. Repetition is the mother of all skills and constant specific concentration achieves results. Coaches know this, teachers know this, and business gurus know this. Specific repetition hones performance and defining the specific is crucial. Refining the specific through repetition is non-negotiable, but what about expectation?

DEFINE AND REFINE

Every teacher recognises the need to be specific: it gives the critical definition of the subject. Sports coaches have drills for everything: from hurdles to strength, from striking skills to tactical skills. The training and educational rehearsals are endless and they vary with every form of education and training regime but how many of us train about expectation? How many of us condition the mind to train the brain?

Russell Worr is a former cycling coach. At one time Russell had a young Jason Kenny is his group. Russ coached and competed and is a student of most sports, including motor racing. In other words, his is a well-rounded brain for preparation in sport. So when Russell invited me to go to the Velodrome soon after it was built, I had no hesitation in accepting. We stood there leaning on the barriers watching the cyclists being put through their paces. My mind wandered around the quite magnificent arena trying to take in all of its splendour. Then Russell asked the question:

'Do bricks and mortar build champions?'

For a few seconds I wondered about this. I paused and thought of the meaning, and then I said:

'Russ, if I were a cyclist and I wanted to compete, I would want to do my training here. This would be the place to train.'

When I look back at our success in producing twenty ageing runners to achieve times of under three hours for the marathon, I could only put it down to expectation. My fortieth and fiftieth birthdays were a result of specific training and expectation. I never ever thought that I wouldn't do it. When Russell Worr asked me the question I had little hesitation in answering. Training at the best possible places raises our expectations.

The future for all of us is how we cope with ageing. Not just in our physical abilities, but how our mind keeps pace with our bodies. Expecting our brains to develop new pathways, neurons, brain cells and synapses need more specifics than just exercise. It needs specific exercise. We need to define these specifics and repeatedly reinforce our expectations. We also need to look at how we absorb the information and learn from our past and from the people who know the answers. We must draw from Mary McDaid, Derek Craynor, Lynn Ward, Sylvia Faucitt and John Higson, interpret their individual secrets and put them together for a collective answer. Our challenge is not to find an answer, but to expect an answer. We have the people, we have the experience and we have the knowledge and now we have a goal.

Our great-grand-daughter Sophia Rose Thorpe is now over one year old. By all predictions and expectations she will live to be over a hundred years of age.

My question now; will she know that she is a hundred years old? If we are to expect a cure then we should expect a prevention? There is no doubt that science recognises that physical exercise is playing a part in rehab and developing new cells even as they are dying. Our children and in our case, our great grand children should know what those exercises are, how they apply them and what we expect them to do. They should know just like they know how to use a computer and their mobile phone. They should know like they know that cardiovascular exercise is good for the heart and weight training builds strength, or protein helps in developing muscle. They should know that a long life is not a given and that we should preserve our mental capacity, work it like we work our muscles, our legs, our arms and our bodies.

We are on the verge of a revolution on extending our physical and mental capacity. The knowledge is there to be used. The science and the start of understanding are there. What we need now is to lower the barriers of entry and raise our expectations and have a vision of the future for the benefits of our children and our children's children.

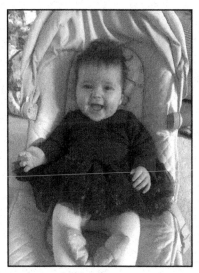

Sophia Rose

"This is not the end, nor is it the beginning of the end, but perhaps it is the end of the beginning."
– Winston Churchill.

26 - ROSETO

In the late 1800s a village called Roseto Valfortore, lay nestling in the rolling landscape of the Apennine Mountains of Southern Italy. The inhabitants in those days were totally dependant on mining the local stone, the most sought after marble in the world. Every able man and boy would trek the four miles to the mine shaft and every able member of the women and elders would work in the surrounding hills harvesting the crops, the only source of nourishment for the villagers.

It was a harsh existence but one that had survived the passage of time. Now after hundreds of years some of the villagers were sensing that changes were coming. The seams of the mines were starting to run out and many were beginning to believe that their future was in doubt.

In 1882 a small group of the townsfolk responded to an invitation to seek work near a town called Bangor in southeast Pennsylvania. The slate mines of Pennsylvania provided a tempting proposition and almost seamless transition for the people of Roseto.

By the early 1900s, almost half of the population of the village in Italy had moved to the city of Bangor. The city's population was made up of mainly German and British people. Not feeling too comfortable with that mix, the Italian immigrants cast their eyes around to look for some alternative. They decided to set up their own little settlement a few miles from the city of Bangor.

No one quite new what triggered this move: perhaps it was the history of generations of the culture of a close-knit community and even a desire for independence. Whatever the reason, the exodus began. Soon the villagers had set up stall with houses, shops and even small factory outlets. The entrepreneurial Italians were starting to build their town. A town they would call Roseto.

By the 1920s, the town had grown to include a church and a town council. The thriving community now provided work in the shops and the expanding factories, employing most of the old and the new generation born on American soil. From the outside and for visitors to the town, this would look just like any other town in the United States. From the inside, however, and looking closer, Roseto, Pennsylvania was unique.

NO ONE DIES OF HEART DISEASE

In 1961, The University of Bangor was hosting a national medical conference and physicians from all over the States attended. The three-day convention consisted of lectures and workshops through the day with time in the evenings to socialise. It was over a pint in the bar that a physician from the University of Oklahoma, Stewart Wolfe, was having a conversation with a local doctor who practised medicine in both Bangor and a local town called Roseto.

'Bangor keeps me busy,' said the local man, 'but I would be out of work if all my patients came from Roseto.'

Not quite sure what he meant, Wolfe asked him to explain. The local doctor went on to say that in the small town of Roseto no one died of illness.

'They all die of old age.'

Not believing what he was hearing, the doctor from the University of Oklahoma asked the local GP to explain further.

'What do you mean? No one is sick in the town of Roseto?'

'I have not had one patient die of heart disease in nearly

ten years', said the doctor. 'In fact no one seems to get sick: I would be redundant if I relied on the people of Roseto.'

Dr Stewart Wolfe by this time was intrigued and asked the local man if he wouldn't mind if he had a closer look at the local medical records. Secretly, he doubted what had been said but what he saw was astonishing.

The records confirmed what the local doctor was saying, so much so that Stewart Wolfe asked the local council if they would object to setting up a full investigation into this phenomenon. He had no doubt that the claims were genuine for the records spoke for themselves. What he wanted to know was how and why.

The first thing that Dr Wolfe did was to recruit doctors and students from his university in Oklahoma. He had already got full cooperation from the Town Council. In fact the locals could not be more helpful. Rooms were even set up in the Town Hall and the family of the Mayor were the first to volunteer to be examined. The results of the investigation were nothing less than amazing and even Dr Wolfe could not unravel the phenomenon of Roseto.

FIRST BREAK ALL THE RULES

Important to the investigation was a colleague of Dr Wolfe, a sociologist called John Brown from his own university in Oklahoma. Between these two experts and all the people they were recruiting they should have been a satisfactory conclusion.

Every possible medical test was conducted: blood tests, ECG and blood pressure and every conceivable question was asked of the volunteers. They weighed, measured and tested, examined their eating habits, and exercise routines, investigated their individual lifestyles and no stone was unturned.

What they found defied everything that they believed in. These people ate everything they fancied: they cooked in animal fat, fried in animal fat and ignored cooking in their traditional olive oil because it was too expensive. Their exercise habits were typically American in that some did, some didn't. Their way of life was no different from any other American in any other town. They smoked, and drank copious amounts of wine. Many of them were overweight and many were obese, but less than half of them needed any form of medication. There was no one on welfare, they had no drug problems and everyone seemed contented and happy with their lot. Dr Stewart Wolfe and Dr John Brown had met their impasse. They had no answer as to why the people of Roseto were as healthy as they were and they did not know how it was happening. The people of Roseto were breaking all the rules and defying the experts, not just Wolfe and Brown, but health experts throughout the world.

Wolfe and Brown where stumped. There were no logical answers, no medical answers and no scientific answers. Not knowing what to do next the doctors decided to go walka-bout. If they could not find the answers the conventional way then they would go the unconventional way.

What they saw was people on the high street stopping and talking to each other, men tipped their hats to the women passing by, shop assistants who knew many of the customers, first names being exchanged and enquiries made about other members of the townsfolk. They noticed families and extended families and how they socialised and how a commu-nity spirit was evident throughout.

The people found reason to visit other families: doors were open and there were barbecues and garden parties. There was always a reason to party, share a beer or a glass of wine. They broke bread together, gossiped together and, in church, prayed together.

The Roseto culture attracted people from all over the country. Every day they would have visitors, some would show just curiosity, some wanted to know more, some would look to settle. Who doesn't want to live longer, be healthier, to be happy?

In time the small town of Roseto grew. The Catholic Church built by the early settlers was joined by another church. Plots of land were bought and new homes sprang up as the population increased. Slowly the culture of the past generation became diluted and bit by bit Roseto became another American town.

These days, when we look at the statistics, we see the same levels of illness, the same percentage of heart conditions as elsewhere. The records show that they have a typical amount of people on welfare and drugs and that obesity is causing people to suffer diabetes.

The small village nestled in the rolling hills of the Apennine Mountains of Southern Italy has lost its influence and the culture that travelled across the world will soon be lost forever.

Over time, the town of Roseto has been absorbed into the body of the United States of America. The tribe mentality, instincts and independence that set the inhabitants apart have all but disappeared. They have in fact become part of the bigger herd, just another statistic.

What happened in that small town in Pennsylvania is a reversal of what has happened with Britain and the European Market. They lost their independence in Roseto and the referendum here has brought it back to Britain. It is ironic that immediately following the exit, Britain had its biggest success ever in the world's largest sporting arena, the Olympic Games.

Are we then seeing the world merge into the five great herds? America, Asia, China, Europe and Africa. All ruled by small groups, or even dictators, pulling the strings of people like the Rosetians, or is there still hope of free thinking, innovation and independence in all of our minds and all of our societies. Only time will tell.

Looking back to those early days, the people living in the village of Roseto Valfortore in Italy were in fact practising the four principles of this book. Their exercise was cultivating the crops, walking to and from the mines. They ate simple food and enjoyed the community of the village. Their mind set was one of peace and happiness and that would probably have prevailed if the seam of the mine had continued.

'Your health comes from within'
Billy Leach

What do you think?

THE END

Lightning Source UK Ltd.
Milton Keynes UK
UKOW06f1124270817
308022UK00002B/9/P